Female Aesthetic Genital Surgery

Editor

CHRISTINE A. HAMORI

CLINICS IN PLASTIC SURGERY

www.plasticsurgery.theclinics.com

October 2022 • Volume 49 • Number 4

ELSEVIER

1600 John F. Kennedy Boulevard ● Suite 1800 ● Philadelphia, Pennsylvania, 19103-2899

http://www.theclinics.com

CLINICS IN PLASTIC SURGERY Volume 49, Number 4
October 2022 ISSN 0094-1298, ISBN-13: 978-0-323-96155-4

Editor: Stacy Eastman
Developmental Editor: Jessica Nicole B. Cañaberal

Clinics in Plastic Surgery (ISSN 0094-1298) is published quarterly by Elsevier Inc., 360 Park Avenue South, New York, NY 10010-1710. Months of issue are January, April, July, and October. Business and Editorial Offices: 1600 John F. Kennedy Blvd., Suite 1800, Philadelphia, PA 19103-2899. Periodicals postage paid at New York, NY and additional mailing offices. Subscription prices are $548.00 per year for US individuals, $1037.00 per year for US institutions, $100.00 per year for US students and residents, $613.00 per year for Canadian individuals, $1234.00 per year for Canadian institutions, $682.00 per year for international individuals, $1234.00 per year for international institutions, $100.00 per year for Canadian and $305.00 per year for international students/residents. To receive student/resident rate, orders must be accompanied by name of affiliated institution, date of term, and the *signature* of program/residency coordinator on institution letterhead. Orders will be billed at individual rate until proof of status is received. Foreign air speed delivery is included in all *Clinics* subscription prices. All prices are subject to change without notice. **POSTMASTER:** Send address changes to *Clinics in Plastic Surgery*, Elsevier Health Sciences Division, Subscription Customer Service, 3251 Riverport Lane, Maryland Heights, MO 63043. **Customer Service: 1-800-654-2452 (US and Canada). From outside of the United States and Canada, call 314-447-8871. Fax: 314-447-8029. E-mail: JournalsCustomerService-usa@elsevier.com (for print support); JournalsOnline-Support-usa@elsevier.com (for online support).**

Reprints. For copies of 100 or more of articles in this publication, please contact the Commercial Reprints Department, Elsevier Inc., 360 Park Avenue South, New York, New York 10010-1710. Tel.: +1-212-633-3874; Fax: +1-212-633-3820; E-mail: reprints@elsevier.com.

Clinics in Plastic Surgery is covered in *Current Contents, EMBASE/Excerpta Medica, Science Citation Index, MEDLINE/PubMed (Index Medicus), ASCA, and ISI/BIOMED.*

Contributors

EDITOR

CHRISTINE A. HAMORI, MD, FACS
Director, Cosmetic Surgery and Skin Spa,
Duxbury, Massachusetts, USA

AUTHORS

RED ALINSOD, MD
Director, Alinsod Institute for Aesthetic
Vulvovaginal Surgery, South Coast
Urogynecology, Inc, Laguna Beach, California,
USA

GARY J. ALTER, MD
Assistant Clinical Professor of Plastic Surgery,
Division of Plastic Surgery, University of
California, Los Angeles, Beverly Hills,
California, USA

SARAH A. APPLEBAUM, MD, MS
Division of Plastic Surgery, Northwestern
University Feinberg School of Medicine,
Chicago, Illinois, USA; Department of Surgery,
University of Maryland Medical Center,
Baltimore, Maryland, USA

EREZ DAYAN, MD
Avance Plastic Surgery, Reno/Tahoe, Nevada,
USA

DAVID GHOZLAND, MD
Angeles, California, USA

**MICHAEL P. GOODMAN, MD, FACOG, IF,
AAACS**
The Labiaplasty and Vaginoplasty Training
Institute of America, Inc, Davis, California,
USA

CHRISTINE A. HAMORI, MD, FACS
Director, Cosmetic Surgery and Skin Spa,
Duxbury, Massachusetts, USA

KRISTI HUSTAK, MD
Clinical Assistant Professor, University of
Texas Medical Branch, Galveston, Texas,
USA; Aesthetic Center for Plastic Surgery,
Houston, Texas, USA

PALLAVI ARCHANA KUMBLA, MD
Aesthetic Center for Plastic Surgery, Houston,
Texas, USA

SOFIA LIU
Sugarland, Texas, USA

OTTO J. PLACIK, MD
Division of Plastic Surgery, Northwestern
University Feinberg School of Medicine,
Chicago, Illinois, USA

MICHAEL A. REED, MD
Cosmetic Gynecologist, Davis, California,
USA

**MARYAM SAHEB-AL-ZAMANI, MA, MD,
FRCSC**
Plastic Surgeon, Private Practice, Toronto,
Ontario, Canada; ICLS Plastic Surgery,
Oakville, Ontario, Canada

LINA TRIANA, MD
Plastic Surgeon, Scientific Director Corpus,
Rostrum Surgery Center, Cali, Valle, Colombia,
South America

ESTEBAN LISCANO
Student, Corpus, Rostrum Surgery Center,
Cali, Valle, Colombia, South America

Contents

care professionals have basic education and tools available to guide patients and to assist clinicians of possible causes and treatment strategies.

Radiofrequency is an effective and safe method for both pelvic floor restoration and nonsurgical labiaplasty. Bipolar radiofrequency with temperature control is more effective than monopolar radiofrequency for volumetric heating of vulvovaginal tissue. Combination of electrical muscle stimulation and radiofrequency can provide combined nonsurgical restoration of the vulvovaginal tissues.

Genital self-image describes the perception of one's genital appearance as being "normal" or "abnormal," and a disharmonious image leads to an increasing number of women seeking esthetic genital surgery each year. The concept of what constitutes "normal" is strongly influenced by the media, cultural norms, and sexual relations. In reality, the extent of normalcy is highly variable and overall patient education regarding extremes of size and shape should be provided to all patients considering surgery. When performed with appropriate training, expertise, and attention to detail in a properly selected patient, esthetic genital surgery is associated with minimal complications or sequelae.

CLINICS IN PLASTIC SURGERY

FORTHCOMING ISSUES

January 2023
Advances and Refinements in Asian Aesthetic Surgery
Lee L.Q. Pu, *Editor*

April 2023
Breast Reconstruction
Neil Tanna, *Editor*

RECENT ISSUES

July 2022
Brow Lift
James E. Zins, *Editor*

April 2022
Plastic Surgery for Men
Douglas S. Steinbrech and Alan Matarasso, *Editors*

SERIES OF RELATED INTEREST

Facial Plastic Surgery Clinics
https://www.facialplastic.theclinics.com/
Otolaryngologic Clinics
https://www.oto.theclinics.com/

THE CLINICS ARE AVAILABLE ONLINE!
Access your subscription at:
www.theclinics.com

Preface
Female Aesthetic Genital Procedures

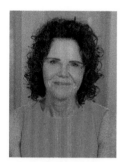

Christine A. Hamori, MD, FACS
Editor

It is a great honor that I have been asked to be the guest editor for the first Female Aesthetic Genital Procedures issue of the *Clinics in Plastic Surgery*. Including this new controversial field among the more traditional plastic surgery topics once and for all validates its existence. In 1998, I performed my first labiaplasty on a young woman encumbered with large labia minora after reading Gary Alter's article on the wedge technique. The surgery went well, but what truly struck me was how happy and confident the patient was afterward.

Now, 25 years later, female aesthetic surgery has expanded with the combined efforts of plastic surgeons and renegade gynecologists who defied American College of Obstetricians and Gynecologists' condemnation of elective female genital procedures. Teaching courses by both specialties are available to train surgeons in proper technique and pelvic anatomy. Residency programs are starting to include exposure to the field as well.

The stigma, however, still exists. Women are still told by well-meaning physicians that aesthetic and functional changes of the vulva from age and pregnancy are immutable. Women want to feel confident about the appearance of their vulvas the same way they do about their breasts and faces. Pubic hair, once a cloak obscuring female genital anatomy, has been lifted. There should be no shame in wanting to look attractive there as well.

Female sexual wellness requires a positive genital self-image, which can be impacted by aberrant anatomy or birth trauma. Who feels confident and sexy with a gaping introitus? Surgical restoration of the muscular anatomy of the introitus and vagina in the form of perineoplasty and vaginoplasty improves the aesthetics and restores sexual function for the woman. These procedures can be performed safely and effectively by properly trained surgeons.

Noninvasive procedures to improve the appearance of the vulva and function of the vagina show promise. The aging process affects the face and vulva in similar ways with fat loss, deflation, and skin laxity. Radiofrequency treatments stimulate collagen to tighten the skin and improve the overall vulvar appearance. Intravaginal treatments with radiofrequency and/or laser have been shown to improve genital syndrome of menopause. Sexual wellness of women at any age can be improved safely and effectively with these noninvasive treatments.

I want to thank the authors for their time and insight into preparing the articles of this issue. I have included not only plastic surgery luminaries in the field of female genital aesthetics but also gynecologists, many of which have been my mentors who specialize in aesthetic and function procedures to improve female sexual wellness. Twenty-five years ago, I would not have thought doing that first labiaplasty would have opened my eyes to this intriguing and rewarding field.

Christine A. Hamori, MD, FACS
Cosmetic Surgery and Skin Spa
113 Tremont Street
Duxbury, MA 02332, USA

E-mail address:
cah@christinehamori.com

Clin Plastic Surg 49 (2022) ix
https://doi.org/10.1016/j.cps.2022.07.003
0094-1298/22/© 2022 Published by Elsevier Inc.

The Evolution of Female Genital Plastic and Cosmetic Surgery: A Cosmetic Gynecologist's Perspective

Michael P. Goodman, MD, FACOG, IF, AAACS

KEYWORDS

- Female genital plastic and cosmetic surgery history • Labiaplasty • Vaginoplasty
- Vulvovaginal esthetics

KEY POINTS

- Labiaplasty began with scattered pediatric and adult patients in the 1970s and 1980s, progressing to more general acceptance as techniques evolved in the 1990s and into the twenty-first century.
- A seminal group of early adaptors and innovators began performing and communicating about genital plastic/cosmetic procedures in the late 1990s and early 2000s.
- Techniques evolved, with multiple studies in the literature reporting on patient satisfaction, complications, and technique evolution in the early years of the twenty-first century.
- Free-standing post-graduate training courses have become available, led by thought leaders in the community.
- Energy-based devices for vaginal and vulvar resurfacing and tissue shrinkage have become available and are evolving. Outcomes are being evaluated.

INTRODUCTION

Mirroring the cosmetic/esthetic surgery performed elsewhere on the body, female genital plastic/cosmetic surgery is performed on normal women. Most of the women presenting to plastic surgeons or cosmetic gynecologists know they are "normal." However, they are not happy with what they experience between their legs, both visually and functionally. I can tell them to "…glory in their normality…" until the cows come home and this will not change how they feel. To quote a patient: "It never bothered my husband, but it was always like "Yuck!" All I know is that what I had I didn't like" (personal communication). It is well-known in the psychological literature that a woman's comfort with her body, especially those parts of her body that have sexual connotations (breasts, belly, vulva, and vagina) directly influences her sexual satisfaction.[1–3] It is curious therefore that over the years in the evolution of this branch of surgical esthetics, there has been such resistance directed against the right of women to change, minimize, lift, and tighten this region.[4–6]

I am an OB/Gyn by training. I ceased delivering babies ~ 20 years ago and discontinued all surgery other than genital aesthetics ~ 10 years ago. While many of my best friends are plastic surgeons (sic), most of the meetings I attend, and my perspective, is that of a cosmetic gynecologist rather than a plastic surgeon, and the comments to follow spring from that perspective.

PERSONAL ANECDOTES FROM THE "EARLY YEARS"

To my knowledge, the earliest labial reductive surgery was the occasional case first performed for functional reasons on pediatric patients. Scattered case reports graced the P.S. and gynecologic literature in the late 1970s and through the 1980s[7–10] and in the early to mid-90s via a variety of

The Labiaplasty and Vaginoplasty Training Institute of America, Inc.™, 4627 Fermi Pl. Suite 110, Davis, CA 95618, USA
E-mail address: Michaelgoodman250@gmail.com

Abbreviations	
Ob/Gyn	Obstetrician/Gynecologist
P.S.	Plastic Surgeon
HPV	human papilloma virus
ABOG	American Board of Obstetrics and Gynecology
ACOG	American College of Obstetricians and Gynecologists
ErYag	Erbium/Yag laser
FGCS	Female Genital Cosmetic Surgery
BBL	Brazlian Butt Lift

pathways, the present "Fathers" in the field of cosmetic gynecology found their personal trailhead. Marco Pelosi II reminisces, "... *In the early 1990s I performed my first purely cosmetic labiaplasty (LP) and hoodectomy. She was 18 year old and I was the physician who delivered her. She was extremely embarrassed with the appearance of her labia minora and hood and had consulted with her gynecologist to fix the problem. He said that there was nothing to be done, and that she should accept her condition—that it was '...ugly...' but perfectly normal. She was living in California, her mother told her to call me and ask for my opinion. She travelled to New Jersey. Her examination confirmed the presence of a very large/hypertrophied labia minora and hood. She asked me if I could do surgery to correct the distorted anatomy, and I said 'no problem.' I did the surgery at my local hospital under general anesthesia. She had an uneventful recovery and the aesthetic results were great. She was very grateful and after all these years she still corresponds with me. The surgery changed her life, she was able to have a normal sexual life without worries about the appearance of her external genitalia and her previously expressed suicidal thoughts were gone... This initial experience made me realize the potential value of aesthetic vulvovaginal surgery and it was responsible for the incorporation of genital surgery to my traditional gynecology practice despite the initial controversial nature of this new field...*" (personal communication).

I had an experience similar to that of Pelosi II described above, when an 18-year-old college student presented for labial reduction. Her "before and after" photos are reproduced in **Fig. 1**, along with the "Thank You" note I received (**Fig. 2**).

In the early 1990s, Gary Alter developed his modified V-wedge design and generously shared it with others, reporting his technique in the literature in 1998.[11] Alter remains a *doyen* in the field and has an international reputation as both a primary and revision surgeon. Red Alinsod got his start in a roundabout way. Being initially trained as a Gyn oncologist and then as a urogynecologist in the late 1980s and early 1990s while in the Air Force at Nellis Air Base outside of Las Vegas, Nevada, Coronel Alinsod first became exposed to laser energy treating vulvar HPV and became aware of the ability of this technology to effect tissue shrinkage. Also, while at Nellis, he was frequently approached for labia minora alteration for comfort and appearance. This was of course Las Vegas, home of the Big Show and Show Girls. He knew the anatomy after performing vulvectomies and exenterations, so it was a short leap to designing labial reductive and vaginal tightening procedures, as he was approached for both of these alterations. After leaving the Air Force in 1994, the next decade of his practice mostly involved urogynecologic procedures, and as the twenty-first century got underway, in addition to performing a handful of LPs, he developed local nerve block procedures which enabled performance of both vulvar and intravaginal procedures on awake patients in an office situation, enabling patients to return home immediately following their procedures. As Alinsod describes, "...*So that is how I got my start. A failed Gyn oncologist, a starter urogynecologist, and finishing up as an esthetic gynecologist. Could not have planned it any better...*" (personal communication).

As an OB/Gyn who had stopped deliveries and had a large Gyn endoscopy, surgical, menopausal, and sexual medicine practice, my first potential LP patient presented in late 1997 with a symptomatic through and through obstetric transection of her right labum, and a robust contralateral side, asking if I could "...fix her flapping...." I designed wedge-like edge excisions of the free edges and a wedge-like reduction of the hypertrophic contralateral side, and it "worked" to the degree that not only was she happy, but she referred a friend who happened to have "bothersome" robust labia. I

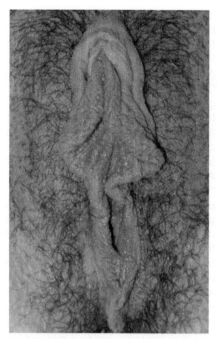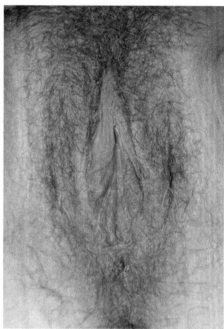

Fig. 1. Before and after V/Y-wedge reduction LP with hood, posterior commissure, and median raphe reduction.

performed a similar procedure, which was also successful. Unfortunately, my third procedure, in early 1999, did not fare as well, and she experienced separation of her wedge repair, but was surprisingly satisfied, as the free edges retracted in relatively esthetic manner, and she had rid herself of her "...elephant ears..." It was around this time that I read Alter's study[11] and learned about subcutaneous "scaffolding" of a wedge repair and subsequent repairs fared better. The first ~ 75 reductive LPs in the late 1990s and early 2000s that I performed were via wedge technique, as linear repairs were at that time problematic secondary to recurrent edge sensitivity. It awaited a technique developed by David Matlock in Los Angeles (personal communication), Pardo S in Chile,[12] and the article from Choi and colleagues,[13] all in the early 2000s which brought the technique of "curvilinear LP" (the term used by Matlock and later popularized as "trim") into the P.S. vernacular. Although he initially held his "new technique" proprietarily quite close to his vest, his use of fine, minimally reactive mostly subcutaneous closure for his "curvilinear" procedures eliminated the frequent edge sensitivity which had compromised the technique since its early days.

In addition, Matlock was among the first surgeons, along with Alinsod, to transform the standard gynecologic "posterior repair" into something quite different: a potentially sexually enhancing vaginal tightening procedure with attention to rebuilding the perineal body. Matlock describes a personal experience: "...While my cosmetic surgery interest started in 1987 with the implementation of liposuction in my practice, in 1996 I applied cosmetic surgical techniques to my vaginal surgical procedures, concerning myself with form, function, and appearance. My first patient was a multiparous woman in her thirties who has stress urinary incontinence and vaginal relaxation. I concerned myself with reconstructing her vaginal floor keeping her relaxation and concern about appearance in mind. After healing, she stated that 'sex is great now;' her husband added that 'it is like having the same wife, but a new woman...' Shortly after they sent me flowers. The rest is history..." (personal communication). Both Goodman and Alinsod describe similar experiences in the early 2000s (personal communications).

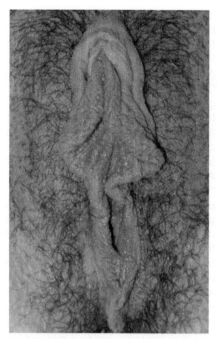

Fig. 2. Letter from patient depicted in Fig. 1.

THE GENESIS OF THE SOCIETIES

Progress in technique development, patient selection, and marketing to the public progressed in fits and starts through the late 1990s and early 2000s. In 2003, Drs Marco Pelosi II and III formed the first society whose mission it was to promote collegiality and exchange of knowledge among gynecologists interested in female genital plastic/cosmetic surgery. At first, the International Society of Cosmetogynecology (ISCG) was a small society whose meetings featured nearly as many faculty members as attendees. Presenters held their cards close to their chests, hesitant to reveal their "secret" techniques. A competing society, "CAVS" (Congress of Aesthetic Vaginal Surgery) was formed by Alinsod around 2004, and the two societies held meetings, often with the number of faculty members outnumbering attendees, and presenters hesitant to describe and reveal their techniques. Goodman, in ~2008 at CAVS was the first presenter to actually describe his surgical technique for reductive LP. Although CAVS faded out as a society at the end of the 2010s, after treading water for several seasons ISCG has rapidly become the major international society at the cutting edge of cosmetic gynecology, drawing faculty and participants from several continents to their annual meetings. In 1998, beginning with meetings in Dubai, the International Cosmetic Gynecology Conference guided by Ayman El Attar MD has also become a major international gathering. Female genital esthetic meetings are now held by many societies worldwide.

The 2010s were distinguished by the development of training programs and increased interest on the part of both women and their providers in providing and consuming genital esthetic procedures. Matlock and Pelosi incorporated genital plastics into their 2 to 3 day training programs in the early/mid 2000s. Alinsod trained his first surgeon ~2005, with Goodman following in 2007 with informal, then formal 2 day programs and Ostrzenski followed suit at approximately the same time. In Europe, the European College of Aesthetic Medicine and Surgery (ECAMS) began trainings in female genital cosmetic surgery in the late 2000s, and Bader, who originally trained for a module of ECAMS (as did Goodman), began his stand-alone courses in the early 2010s, with Kuzlik, Seifeldin, and others in Europe, Asia, and the Middle East, offering training programs beginning in the past several years. With the addition of two textbooks on the subject,[14,15] short postgraduate programs, and the several 2 to 3 day hands-on courses now offered worldwide, there is presently no excuse for the surgeon untrained in his or her residency in esthetic LP and "vaginal tightening" to undertake esthetic reductive LP or functional vaginal tightening reconstructions. The residency program directors, the ABOG, and the ACOG continue, in my opinion, to drag their feet. OB/Gyn residents for the most part continue to graduate without either training in plastic surgery technique, understanding of the emotional pain and functional issues women with "robust endowment" experience, and receive no meaningful training in genital esthetics including esthetic LP. As a result, as women are approaching their "OB/Gyn" at increasing rates for vulvar reduction procedures, those of us who include revision surgery of poorly conceived procedures in our repertoire are seeing an uptick in requests from revision from women with amputation or neuropathic pain from the placement of sutures inconsistent with P.S. principles. Women as well seek our services after undergoing site-specific pelvic floor repairs by skilled Gyn or Urogyn surgeons where sexual issues involving her vaginal relaxation were never part of pre-op discussion or surgical planning.

The 2000s and 2010s proceeded surgically with many bells and whistles, but all attached to the same vehicle: "linear/trim" and "wedge" procedures remain King and Queen (or Queen and King...), although the technically more difficult procedure of de-epithelialization is adopted by some. Many have written regarding embellishments designed to make these two stalwarts more reproducible, safer, and better,[16,17] and the "subspecialty" became richer with their upgrades. The major change, beginning in the early 2010s, was the introduction of so-called energy-based devices (EBDs) into both clinical practice and the vernacular. Unfortunately, in my opinion, the term "Vaginal Rejuvenation" became misappropriated as the Flagship for this novel addition to a field that had heretofore been dominated by surgical approaches.

WHAT "Laser VAGINAL REJUVENATION" ORIGINALLY MEANT

In 2003, Matlock, whose degrees include both an MD and an MBA, attempted to patent his new vaginal tightening procedure, in which he used a touch laser fiber *as his cutting tool*. He called his new procedure "Laser Vaginal Rejuvenation." The term was further promoted at meetings and in the literature in the mid-2000s by Miklos and Moore in Atlanta,[18] who incorporated esthetic gynecology in their large international urogynecology practice. The term was bandied about at meetings, again meaning a *surgical* vaginal tightening procedure using a touch laser fiber as a cutting tool. Around the same time researchers in Israel, Italy and elsewhere began experimenting with novel applications for laser energy, and platforms delivering both ErYag and fractional CO2 (FrCO2) laser energy previously used for skin resurfacing and regeneration on other areas of the body, most notably the face, were envisioned for novel areas of the body, notably the female genitalia. Hand pieces were developed to deliver this energy onto the vaginal mucosal epithelium, and prototypes were investigated in several countries. The companies wishing to place as many of these units with newly minted genitally friendly hand pieces as possible, adapted the old phrase "Vaginal Rejuvenation" as their moniker. "Laser Vaginal Rejuvenation" was now reimagined, with the laser energy here defocused, rather than the focused cutting tool used by Matlock.

Vaginal rejuvenation (VRJ), a marketing tool and social media term rather than a one defined in the medical nomenclature, has become an umbrella term used to describe a range of esthetic and functional procedures that correct and restore the optimal structure of the vagina and surrounding tissues. However, what, really, does VRJ mean?? On the one end of the spectrum lie noninvasive strategies that serve as a first-line approach to improving vaginal atrophy and dryness, such as lubricants and hormone replacement medications and/or Kegel exercises aiming to strengthen the pelvic floor muscles. On the other end, gynecologic or plastic surgeons perform invasive procedures such as LP to alter the labia minora and majora and the folds of skin surrounding the clitoris or vaginoplasty (VP), which involves surgery aimed at attenuating and supporting the pelvic floor. The term, "VP" is a misnomer. Not found in the medical literature and even though quite descriptive, it really refers to the surgical procedure of levatorplasty which, if care is not taken to avoid excessive traction on nerves within the levator musculature can lead to an increased incidence of dyspareunia.[19] This led to reimagining the operation under local anesthesia by Alinsod, and then Goodman, with an awake patient who can alert her surgeon to levator or perineal body sutures which are at once painful on tightening. With the awake patient, the potentially errantly placed suture may be safely repositioned.

THE ADVENT OF ENERGY-BASED DEVICES: GOING BEYOND SURGERY AND ESTABLISHING "GENITAL ESTHETICS"

Nonsurgical vulvovaginal therapy, whether via various radiofrequency (RF) or laser devices, has been one of the fastest growing areas in plastic surgery and urogynecology over the past 10 years.[20,21] We see marketing for "Vaginal Rejuvenation" in

medical spas, gynecology, plastic surgery, and dermatology offices with little explanation regarding what that term actually entails and truly accomplishes. As both laser and RF energy is, as they say, only "skin deep" any effect on vaginal tightening is superficial and temporary, not involving reanastomosis of muscles or fascia, or excision of adynamic post-parturition scar tissue. The literature seems to be clear that, with a three treatment regimen of procedures ~ 1 month apart, increased mucosal flexibility and subjective vaginal support is noticed by patients for 3 to 6 months, but all studies suffer from a lack of the sham group and any follow-up past 6 months, and no studies compared the results at alternative energy settings (Watt; Hz; Joules).[21–24] Results must be maintained by "touch-up" re-treatments at least every 6 to 9 months. At ~$800 to 1000 per session, over time this can be both time-consuming and expensive, since unlike surgery, positive effects are temporary and must be maintained. The patient must make a trip to her health care practitioner three times over 2 months for benefits that do not seem to last well greater than 6 to 9 months.

There are data in regard to the use of pixilated FrCO2 pulsed laser for stress urinary incontinence (SUI) and improvement of vulvovaginal atrophy associated with genitourinary syndrome of menopause. Vaginal FrCO2 has been found to be effective for mild-to-moderate SUI over a follow-up period of 1 year, according to a variety of objective and subjective parameters.[25–27] FrCO2 has been found effective for up to 3 years using a treatment protocol of therapy sessions monthly X 3 to 4, with annual "touch-ups." Intravaginal therapy with mono or bipolar RF apparatus such as ThermiVa and others have been widely touted, but evidence-based literature is scant and poorly powered and with very short follow-up.[21–24,28] Although there is a lot of money to be made by temporizing with EBDs for vaginal tightening, adding a minimally invasive procedure such as FrCO2 laser or RF to a surgical VP for the temporary nonsurgical treatment of SUI has benefits, although it must be regularly repeated every 1+ years.

HOW DO ENERGY-BASED DEVICES FIT IN TO THE EVOLUTION OF "GENITAL PLASTICS..?"

EBDs certainly have a place in this evolution. Many women wish to temporize as relates to vaginal tightening to improve coital friction and to try an energy-based therapy to see if they can avoid a surgical procedure. I have no quarrel with this approach, so long as clinicians are honest with their patients regarding the number of visits, minimalistic "tightening" results and the expected length of these results as they relate to improved coital friction, which is certainly no more than 6 to 12 months, and may be as little as 3 months. In their systematic review, Preminger and colleagues[29] found that most of the studies resulted in mild to no adverse side effects. However, there is a large gap in level I evidence and no long-term (>6 months follow-up) studies in the literature regarding the efficacy of RF-based devices for both improving vagina tightness and treating urinary incontinence.

FINAL THOUGHTS

Evolution involves all species. Here, we have multiple interests: the patient, the provider, and the ethics governing the interaction of these interested parties. Does female genital plastic/cosmetic surgery and therapy with EBDs pass the ethical sniff test? Goldstein and Goldstein[30] weighed in years ago, speaking of the tenets of medical ethics: patient autonomy, nonmaleficence, beneficence, justice, and veracity and concluded that indeed the field of FGCS did pass the sniff test, provided that ethical guidelines were followed. Is it ethical to perform an operation viewed by our patients as inherently cosmetic without requisite training? Is it ethical to tell our patient, in the absence of reproducible evidence that "...we will try laser (or RF) and if that does not work we can always do surgery..." without a thorough explanation of all of the parameters?

In her fascinating article,[31] Rodrigues posits that "...the increased attention and demand for these two surgeries (LP; VP) signifies a contemporary (re)deployment of biopower aimed at making the vagina more useful. In particular, I suggest that LP introduces esthetics as another dimension of disciplinary control, whereas VP reaffirms that the value of the vagina is fixed in its receptive capability. Taken together, I argue, VP and LP are indicative of a deployment of biopolitics in service of the creation of the 'optimal' vagina."

From general anesthesia to local anesthesia, from hospital to properly equipped office, and from nomadic surgeons wandering in the figurative desert to trained surgeons communicating with each other at Congresses and via evidence-based publications, the "subspecialty" progresses. Techniques are reimagined and refined. Outcomes are reported and analyzed. Unfortunately, societies such as ACOG and ABOG continue, as the proverbial ostrich, to invalidate vulvovaginal esthetics as part of the purview of gynecologic surgeons,[32,33] and we continue to see the tragedy of "unintentional avoidable female genital mutilations" performed by well-meaning gynecologic surgeons untrained in the "Rules" or the nuances of FCGS, and women are harmed.

Women (and men!) certainly have many different body parts which may protrude, sag, fold, hang, discolor, and age in ways unappealing to their "wearers." The most important question, *are we helping our patients*, appears, from the evidence-based literature, to be a qualified "yes," as the field evolves. Plastic surgeons with requisite training perform LPs and cosmetic perineoplasties. Cosmetic gynecologists perform both plus more invasive levatorplasty/VP procedures. However, as Sasson and colleagues have discovered in a niftily conceived study of women's attitudes regarding genital FGCS,[32] a stigma persists regarding alterations involving the organs "...down there." Although it is OK to conceive of and accomplish esthetic procedures involving bodily areas with sexual connotations such as breasts and bellies, attitudes regarding genital alterations remain mired in the shame-based and puritanical attitudes of our forebears toward female genitalia. It still is not "right," not something to be openly shared (as is breast reduction or augmentation; rhinoplasty; abdominoplasty; BBL; and so forth). So, as procedures have evolved, as sharing of knowledge has evolved, and as women's decisions to contemplate revisions "...down there" have evolved, the decision to share these surgical concerns and discussions perhaps has not, and to some extent these procedures remain secret, to be discussed only between patient and practitioner. As such, our patients put an amazing amount of *trust* in their practitioner, and it is the practitioner's *responsibility* to not betray this trust.

CLINICS CARE POINTS

- Surgeons performing surgical esthetic/functional labiaplasty or vaginovulvar procedures designed to produce increased friction for sexual enhancement should be specifically trained in these procedures in residency or a stand-alone program or to be "Grandfathered" by performing a reasonably large number of procedures.

- Clinicians should emphasize to their patients that vulvovaginal therapy with energy-based devices has temporary results, which may be inferior to results obtained with surgical procedures for the same presentation.

DISCLOSURE

The author received no aid, financial or in-kind, from any outside source in the preparation of this article.

REFERENCES

1. Pujols Y, Meston CM, Seal BN. The association between sexual satisfaction and body image in women. J Sex Med 2010;7:905–16.
2. Shick VR, Calabrese SK, Rima BN, et al. Genital appearance dissatisfaction: implications for women' genital image self-consciousness, sexual esteem, sexual satisfaction, and sexual risk. Psychol Women Q 2010;34:394–404.
3. Berman L, Windecker M. The relationship between women's genital self-image and female. sexual function: a national survey. Curr Sex Heal Rep 2008;5:199–207.
4. Tiefer L. Female genital cosmetic surgery: Freakish or inevitable? Analysis from medical marketing, bioethics, and feminist theory. Fem Psychol 2008;18:466–79.
5. Liao LM, Creighton SM. Requests for cosmetic genitoplasty: how should healthcare providers respond? BMJ 2007;334:1090–2.
6. Iglesia CB. Cosmetic gynecology and the elusive quest for the "perfect" vagina. Obstet Gynecol 2012;119:1083–4.
7. Hodgkinson DJ, Hait G. Aesthetic vaginal labiaplasty. Plast Reconstr Surg 1984;74:414–6.
8. Rubayi S. Aesthetic vaginal labioplasty. Plast Reconstr Surg 1985;75:608.
9. Honore LH, O'Hara KE. Benign enlargement of the labia minora: report of two cases. Eur J Obstet Gynecol Reprod Biol 1978;8:61–4.
10. Chavis WM, LaFeria JJ, Niccolini R. Plastic repair of elongated hypertrophic labia minora. A case report. J Reprod Med 1989;34:3737–45.
11. Alter GJ. A new technique for aesthetic labia minora reduction. Ann Plast Surg 1998;40:287–90.
12. Pardo J, Sola P, Ricci P, et al. Laser labiaplasty of the labia minora. Int J Gynecol Obstet 2005;93:38–43.
13. Choi HY, Kin KT. A new method for aesthetic reduction of the labia minora. Plast Reconstr Surg 2000; 105:419–24.
14. Goodman MP, editor. Female genital plastic and cosmetic surgery. 1st edition. Chichester (UK): John Wiley & Sons, Ltd; 2016.
15. Hamori C, Banwell P, Alinsod R. Female genital cosmetic surgery: concepts, classification and techniques. 1st edition. New York: Thieme; 2019.
16. Kelishadi SS, Elston JB, Rao AJ, et al. Posterior wedge resection: a more aesthetic labiaplasty. Aesthet Surg J 2013;33(6):847–53.
17. Cao Y, Li Q, Li F, et al. Aesthetic labia minora reduction with combined wedge-edge resection: a modified approach of labiaplasty. Aesthet Plast Surg 2015;39(1):36–42.
18. Miklos J, Moore R. Vaginal reconstruction and rejuvenation surgery: is there data to support improved sexual function? Am J Cosmet Surg 2012;29:97–113.
19. Miklos JR, Kohli N, Moore R. Levatorplasty release and reconstruction of rectovaginal septum using allogenic dermal graft. Int Urogynecol J Pelvic Floor Dysfunct 2002;13(1):44–6.
20. Desai SA, Kroumpouzos G, Sadik N. Vaginal rejuvenation: from scalpel to wands. Int J Womens Dermatol 2019;5(2):79–84.
21. Qureshi AA, Tenenbaum MM, Myckatyn TM. Nonsurgical vulvovaginal rejuvenation with radiofrequency and laser devices: a literature review and comprehensive update for aesthetic surgeons. Aesthet Surg J 2018;38:302.
22. Krychman M, Rowan CG, Allan BB, et al. Effect of single-treatment, surface-cooled radiofrequency therapy on vaginal laxity and female sexual function: the VIVEVE I randomized controlled trial. J Sex Med 2017;14(2):215–25.
23. Millheiser LS, Pauls RN, Herbst SJ, et al. Radiofrequency treatment of vaginal laxity after vaginal delivery: nonsurgical vaginal tightening. J Sex Med 2010; 7(9):3088–95.
24. Alinsod RM. Transcutaneous temperature controlled radiofrequency for orgasmic dysfunction. Lasers Surg Med 2016;48(7):641–5. https://doi.org/10.1002/lsm.22537.
25. Alcaly M, Ben Ami M, Greenshpun A, et al. Fractional-pixel CO 2 laser treatment in patients with urodynamic stress urinary incontinence: 1-year F levatorplasty release and reconstruction of rectovaginal septum using allogenic dermal graftollow-up lasers. J Surg Med 2021;53(7):960–7.
26. Behnia-Willison F, Nguyen TT, Mahamadi B, et al. Fractional CO2 laser for the treatment of Stress Urinary Incontinence. Eur J Obstet Gynecol Reprod Biol X 2019;1:100004.
27. Gonzalez Isaza p, Jaguszewski K, Cardona JL, et al. Long-term effect of thermoablative fractional CO 2 laser treatment as a novel approach to urinary incontinence management in women with genitourinary syndrome of menopause. Int Urogynecol J 2018;29(2):211–5.
28. Karcher C, Sadick N. Vaginal Rejuvenation using energy-based devices. Int J Womens Dermatol 2016;2(3):85–8.
29. Preminger M, Kurtzman JS, Dayan B. A systematic review of nonsurgical vulvovaginal restoration devices: an evidence-based examination of safety and efficacy. Plast Reconstr Surg 2020;146(5):552e–64e.
30. Goodman MP, Bachman G, Johnson C, et al. Is elective vulvar plastic surgery ever warranted, and what screening should be conducted preoperatively? J Sex Med 2007;4:269–76.
31. Rodrigues S. From vaginal exception to exceptional vagina: the biopolitics of female genital cosmetic surgery. Sexualities 2012;15(7):778–94.
32. Practice Guideline. Elective female genital cosmetic surgery: ACOG Committee Opinion, Number 795. Obstet Gynecol 2020;135(1):e36–42.
33. Sasson DC, Hamori CA, Placik OJ. Labiaplasty: the stigma persists. Aesthet Surg J 2021;9:sjab335.

Anatomical Changes of the Vulva Due to Childbirth and Aging

Kristi Hustak, MD[a,*], Pallavi Archana Kumbla, MD[a], Sofia Liu[b]

KEYWORDS

- Hormonal changes of female reproductive system • Pelvic organ prolapse • Vulvovaginal atrophy
- Vulvar anatomy • Pregnancy-induced changes of female reproductive system

KEY POINTS

- Changes occur in the female reproductive system throughout life.
- Key changes occur during major times of hormonal shifts such as puberty, pregnancy, and menopause.
- Pelvic organ prolapse can be classified into four subgroups.
- These changes can cause severe symptoms for women and may require nonsurgical or surgical intervention depending on severity.

INTRODUCTION

The female reproductive system is composed of several organs.[1] These include the ovaries, fallopian tubes, uterus, uterine cervix, vagina, and vulva. The vulva consists of the labia majora, labia minora, clitoris, vulvar vestibule, urethral meatus, and vaginal orifice. The vagina is a fibromuscular organ that extends from the vaginal introitus to the uterine cervix and is composed of an anterior and posterior wall. The anterior wall borders the posterior bladder, whereas the posterior wall borders the anterior rectal wall. Within the vulva, the labia majora border the labia minora. The vulvar vestibule contains the urethra and the vaginal opening. As females age, there are physiologic changes that occur within all of these organs. The most dramatic effects occur during key times of hormonal shifts such as puberty, pregnancy, and menopause.

ANATOMY OF THE FEMALE REPRODUCTIVE SYSTEM

To understand the changes that occur over time, one must understand the embryologic development of the female reproductive system.[2] The vaginal epithelium derives from the endoderm of the urogenital sinus, whereas the fibromuscular wall develops from the mesenchymal layer. The vaginal lumen forms from the vaginal plate which derives from the sinovaginal bulb. In regard to external genitalia, this is not fully differentiated until week 12. Estrogen plays a key role in this process and is responsible for feminization of the external genitalia. Growth of the phallus is halted and becomes the clitoris. The urogenital folds become the labia minora. The labioscrotal folds become the labia majora and mons. The mons, labia majora, and clitoris age like skin in other areas of the body as they are made up of stratified, keratinized epithelium. The vulvar vestibule, labia minora, introitus, hymen, and urethral orifice contain nonkeratinized skin.

PHYSIOLOGIC CHANGES OF THE FEMALE REPRODUCTIVE SYSTEM THROUGHOUT LIFE

During infancy and childhood, the vulva and vagina are influenced by maternal estrogen that remains following birth. The labia majora and labia minora are developed as a result and the vaginal mucosa contains glycogen. In addition, *Lactobacillus*

a Aesthetic Center for Plastic Surgery, 12727 Kimberley Lane, Suite 300, Houston, TX 77024, USA; b 4110 Turtle Trails Lane, Sugarland, TX 77479, USA
* Corresponding author.
E-mail address: kristihustakmd@gmail.com

Clin Plastic Surg 49 (2022) 429–433
https://doi.org/10.1016/j.cps.2022.06.005

becomes present within 24 hours. Estrogen levels decrease after 4 weeks and as a result the vaginal epithelium becomes thinner. Similarly, the labia majora, mons, and vulvar skin thin.[3]

By puberty (ages 8 to 13), estrogen levels increase. The results of this include a thickened vaginal epithelium. The labia majora and mons increase in subcutaneous fat. The vulva also thickens and the clitoris enlarges. The introitus increases in diameter. At this time as well, vaginal secretions become more acidic. Although menstruation does increase the pH of the vagina transiently, acidity is maintained by several lactic acid producing species, including four predominant types of *Lactobacillus*.[3]

These changes are maintained until pregnancy occurs. During this time, there is an increase in total blood volume. Cardiac output increases as early as 5 weeks and by 24 weeks is increased by approximately 45% in a singleton pregnancy.[4] This is coupled by a decrease in peripheral vascular resistance.[5] This leads to engorgement and distention of the vulva and to the hyperpigmentation seen in the vulva and vagina. In addition, progesterone levels increase leading to distensibility of the venous system which can cause varicosities. Varicosities are common, accounting for 18% to 22% of pregnant women, with the majority (91%) occurring in women that have had more than two term pregnancies.[6,7] Varicosities usually resolve by 6 weeks postpartum but can persist in 4% to 8% of patients.[8] The vaginal musclar sling strengthens and thickens (hypertrophy was essentially to describe this phenomenon) to prepare for childbirth while the connective tissue layers of the vagina, perineum, and vulva relax. These changes can lead to a feeling of fullness and heaviness, and for some women, pain. These symptoms can worsen as the fetus moves deeper in the dependent pelvis and restricts blood flow. By the time of delivery, the vaginal and perineal musculature has relaxed. This in combination with vaginal rugae flattening allows the vaginal tract to dilate to accommodate the passage of the baby. The introitus is larger after vaginal delivery.[3] Although the anatomy of the female reproductive tract may return to its norm by 3 months, with subsequent parity, these changes may not completely normalize. The dilation and stretch of the introitus, the elongation and hanging of the labia majora, and the stretch of the pelvic floor muscles may persist in some women and become symptomatic.

VAGINAL LAXITY

Among parous women, reports of vaginal laxity are more prevalent among spontaneous vaginal births versus cesarean sections. This risk is also increased by the use of instrumentation in vaginal delivery.[9] Routine episiotomies are common and there is no clear data, to date, on whether episiotomies have an impact on pelvic floor relaxation or pelvic organ prolapse in the long term. There however seems to be a linear relationship between the degree of perineal laceration and postpartum dyspareunia.[10] Women report an incidence of vaginal laxity following childbirth 24% to 48%, however, nulliparous women also report vaginal laxity 4.8% of the time.[11,12] In this latter patient population, coitus is likely a contributing factor. This is supported by the clusters of complaints in younger patients in their prime sexual years.[11–14] Further compounding the issue of vaginal laxity is that these issues are frequently underreported. According to a 2010 study, 80% of women failed to mention symptoms of vaginal laxity to their gynecologist.[15]

Vaginal laxity, or excessive looseness, is a broad term that is ill-defined and its subjective nature makes it difficult to study. Women often complain of decreased sensation with vaginal penetration, increased pelvic pressure, bulging, fullness, or vaginal flatus. Although one study has correlated complaints of vaginal laxity to objective measurements and imaging of pelvic organ prolapse, others have found no correlation.[9,11] Body mass index (BMI) has no correlation on complaints of vaginal laxity but does increase incidence of clinical pelvic organ prolapse.[9,14]

PELVIC ORGAN PROLAPSE

Pelvic organ prolapse is defined as herniation of the anterior vaginal wall, posterior vaginal wall, uterus, or vaginal apex into the vagina. Prolapse can involve one or all of these structures. Although pregnancy is the most common risk factor for pelvic organ prolapse, other factors include Hispanic or Caucasian ethnicity, age, connective tissue disorders, family history of prolapse, chronic cough, constipation, heavy lifting, and hysterectomy or prior prolapse surgery. Normal support of the pelvis is provided by a network of muscular slings, ligaments, and fascia to support the pelvic floor structures such as the bladder, urethra, uterus, vagina, and rectum. The paired levator ani muscles (iliococcygeus, pubococcygeus, and puborectalis) and the ischiococcygeus muscles are the main muscles of support (**Fig. 1**). The levator ani muscles can become stretched or injured as one ages and with childbirth and become more vertically oriented which opens the vagina and leads to prolapse (**Fig. 2**).[16] Muscle mass often decreases as one ages, compounding the problem. As the perineum

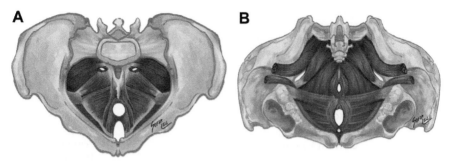

Fig. 1. (*A*) Anatomy of female pelvic floor musculature. (*B*) Anatomy of female pelvic floor musculature. (*Courtesy of* Sofia Liu, Houston, TX.)

loses its tone, hymenal remnants and the lower vaginal vault mucosa can become more visible at rest, leading to change in both the appearance and function of the lower tract. Levator ani hyperdistensibility has the strongest association clinically with complaints of vaginal laxity.[11]

Pelvic organ prolapse can be categorized into four groups, described in 1972 by the Baden–Walker classification (**Table 1**). In grade 0, there is no prolapse. In grade 1, there is descent halfway to the hymen. In grade 2, there is descent to the hymen. In grade 3, there is descent halfway past the hymen. Finally, in grade 4, there is maximal possible descent for each site.[16] This has been further modified in 1996 by the Quantitative pelvic organ prolapse (POP) into four stages (see **Table 1**): stage 0, no prolapse; stage II, greater than 1 cm above the hymen; stage III is 1 cm or less proximal or distal to the plane of the hymenal ring; and stage III is greater than 1 cm below the plane of the hymenal ring but no more than 2 cm less than the total vaginal length. Stage IV is complete eversion of the lower vaginal tract. To fully delineate prolapse and its degree, a pelvic examination must be performed. Based on the grade of prolapse, several options may exist for resolution, including observation, Kegel exercises, pessaries, or surgical intervention.

VULVOVAGINAL ATROPHY AND MENOPAUSE

Finally, in the later stages of life, vulvovaginal atrophy may occur during menopause. Menopause typically occurs around the age of 50 when the menstrual cycle ceases for 12 consecutive months. Vulvovaginal atrophy, or more aptly, genitourinary syndrome of menopause (GSM), is due to the decreased levels of estrogen and occurs in 4% of premenopausal women and 47% in the postmenopausal group.[17] Estrogen functions to keep the vaginal mucosa thick, lubricated, and elastic with increased blood flow. As it decreases, women experience a drier, inelastic vagina that is often paler in color than its younger pink hue. The vaginal vault shrinks in both length and width. Thinning of mucosa can cause chronic burning and itching, leading to dyspareunia. Additional changes in the vulvovaginal anatomy typically seen include declining pubic hair, volume loss of the labia majora and mons, and indistinct and lighter labia minora. Vaginal secretions decrease and vaginal pH increases. Periurethral tissue thins. This leads to increased urinary tract infections due to the increased prevalence of enteric species and bacterial vaginosis from pH shifts. Other issues such as lichen sclerosis also can develop with vulvovaginal atrophy.[3]

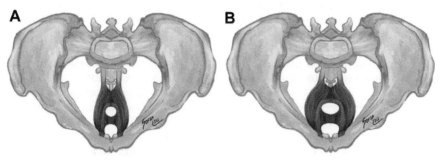

Fig. 2. (*A*) Levator ani musculature in the nulliparous patient. (*B*) Levator ani musculature stretch seen in aging and postpartum. (*Courtesy of* Sofia Liu, Houston, TX.)

Table 1
Baden–Walker grading and POP-Q staging of pelvic organ prolapse

Baden–Walker System		POP-Q Classification	
Grade		Stage	
0	No prolapse	0	No prolapse
1	Descent halfway to the hymen	I	>1 cm above the hymen
2	Descent to the hymen	II	<1 cm proximal or distal to the plane of the hymen
3	Descent half way past the hymen	III	>1 cm below the hymen plane but less than 2 cm of the TVL
4	Eversion of the genital tract	IV	Eversion of the lower genital tract

POP-Q, Pelvic Organ Prolapse-Questionnaire; TVL, Total Vaginal Length

SUMMARY

In summary, physiologic and anatomic changes occur in the female reproductive system from birth to menopause and are directly influenced by hormonal levels. These changes can lead to laxity of the female reproductive organs that can cause significant symptoms in women. These symptoms are often underreported and are a prime area for increased research and inquest to further define the scope of the problem, implement surgical and nonsurgical techniques to improve it, and subsequently advance the overall quality of life in those to which it impacts.

CLINICS CARE POINTS

- Pregnant women should be counseled of the changes in the female genitalia that will occur during pregnancy and that these changes may not return to their prepregnancy state.

- When a patient presents for clinical evaluation, a thorough history and evaluation of symptoms is critical to avoid missing a diagnosis of pelvic organ prolapse.

- Physical examination including a complete pelvic examination should be performed to determine the grade of prolapse to determine the proper intervention required.

- Patients should be educated on nonsurgical and surgical techniques suited to correct their symptoms.

ACKNOWLEDGMENTS

Fully funded it through my private practice (the aesthetic center for plastic surgery)

DISCLOSURE

The authors of this article have no commercial or financial conflicts of interest.

REFERENCES

1. Rosner J, Samardzic T, Sarao MS. Physiology, female reproduction. In: StatPearls. Treasure Island (FL): StatPearls Publishing; 2021.
2. PowerShow. Development of female genital system. 2021. Available at: https://www.powershow.com/viewfl/3f24a4-MzZjN/DEVELOPMENT_OF_FEMALE_GENITAL_SYSTEM_powerpoint_ppt_presentation. Accessed December 21, 2021.
3. Farage M, Maibach H. Lifetime changes in the vulva and vagina. Arch Gynecol Obstet 2005;273(4): 195–202.
4. Hunter S, Robson SC. Adaptation of the maternal heart in pregnancy. Heart 1992;68(12):540–3.
5. Sanghavi M, Rutherford JD. Cardiovascular physiology of pregnancy. Circulation 2014;130(12): 1003–8.
6. Gavrilov SG. Vulvar varicosities: diagnosis, treatment, and prevention. Int J Women's Health 2017; 9:463–75.
7. Fassiadis N. Treatment for pelvic congestion syndrome causing pelvic and vulvar varices. Int Angiol 2006;25:1–3.
8. Bell D, Kane PB, Liang S, et al. Vulvar varices: an uncommon entity in surgical pathology. Int J Gynecol Pathol 2007;26:99–101.
9. Talab S. Correlates of vaginal laxity symptoms in women attending a urogynelogical clinic in Saudi Arabia. Int J Gynecol Obstet 2019;145: 278–82.
10. AbdoolZ Thakar R, Sultan AH. Postpartum female sexual function. Eur J Obstet Gynecol Reprod Biol 2009;145:133–7.

11. Dietz HP, Stankiewicz M, Atan IK, et al. Vaginal laxity: what does this symptom mean? Int Urogynecol J 2018;29:723–8.

12. Durnea CM, Khashan AS, Kenny LC, et al. An insight into pelvic floor status in nulliparous women. Int Urogynecol J 2014;25:337–45.

13. Shifren JL, Monz BU, Russo PA, et al. Sexual problems and distress in United States women: prevalence and correlates. Obstet Gynecol 2008;112:970–8.

14. MacLennan AH, Taylor AW, Wilson DH, et al. The prevalence of pelvic floor disorders and their relationship to gender, age, parity and mode of delivery. BJOG 2000;107:1460–70.

15. Millheiser L, Kingsberg S, Pauls R. A cross-sectional survey to assess the prevalence and symptoms associated with laxity of the vaginal introitus [Abstract 206]. Presented at: ICS Annual Meeting; Toronto, Ontario, Canada. August 23–27, 2010.

16. Iglesia CB. Pelvic organ prolapse surgery. JAMA 2013;309(19):2045.

17. Mac Bride MB, Rhodes DJ, Shuster LT. Vulvovaginal atrophy. Mayo Clin Proc 2010;85(1):87–94.

The Aesthetic Genital Consultation
Inquiry to Scheduling

Christine A. Hamori, MD

KEYWORDS

- Labiaplasty • Vaginoplasty • Perineoplasty • Labia minora reduction • Women's sexual health
- Vaginal laxity • Gaping introitus

KEY POINTS

- Labiaplasty consultation and examination.
- Validated questionnaires in the evaluation of female aesthetic genital patients.
- Evaluation of vaginal laxity.
- Managing patients interested in labiaplasty, clitoral hood reduction, or labia majora reduction.
- Informed consent in labiaplasty and vaginoplasty.

The popularity of aesthetic genital procedures has increased exponentially over the past 10 years. The trend is thought to increase in 2022 due to the popularity of cycling and athleisure.[1]

Plastic surgeons and more recently gynecologists are seeing an influx of women interested in treatment options to improve the esthetics of their genitalia. In addition, women want to improve sexual function, which is often affected by pregnancy and aging. The provider needs to understand the mindset of these patients and effectively navigate the consultation with the goal of assessing the patients' needs and wants regarding aesthetic genital procedures.

HOW DO PATIENTS FIND YOU?

Unlike more traditional plastic surgical inquiries such as breast enhancement or abdominoplasty, female genital concerns are still considered taboo and rarely promoted on social media except perhaps by the likes of the Kardashian sisters. Patients usually research treatment of "large labia minora" or "vaginal laxity" under the presumed cloak of anonymity of the Internet. The 2 landing points for the inquiries are physician Web sites and patient community portals like Real Self, which permit the display of genital before and after photographs.

Web site content is best placed under a separate category from other body contouring procedures to enable patients and search engines the ability to discover information on female aesthetic genital procedures. A dedicated micro Web site on the topic helps keep sensitive-to-some information isolated yet available to those who are interested in aesthetic genital procedures. Simple labeled anatomic diagrams help patients understand their specific areas of concern. Female genital anatomy is complicated for patients to understand when compared with other body parts such as the face, body, and breast.

Patient communities like Real Self provide a haven for those interested in genital aesthetic procedures because genital before and after photographs are not censored as they are on social media. Women share their opinions and surgical journeys in tremendous detail allowing potential patients to familiarize themselves with the procedures and the recovery process. It behooves surgeons to contribute photographs and submit content to such sites where patients interested in such procedures may be searching. Before and after pictures should be standardized (one standing before and after and one lithotomy before and after [**Fig. 1**]).

Cosmetic Surgery and Skin Spa, 113 Tremont Street, Duxbury, MA 02332, USA
E-mail address: cah@christinehamori.com

Clin Plastic Surg 49 (2022) 435–445
https://doi.org/10.1016/j.cps.2022.06.006
0094-1298/22/© 2022 Elsevier Inc. All rights reserved.

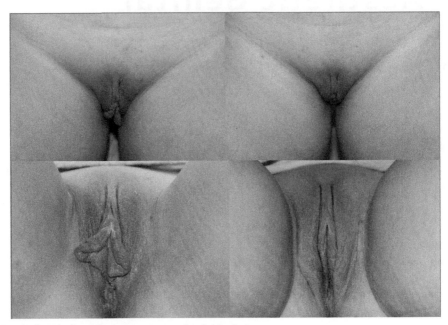

Fig. 1. A 35 y/o female 8 weeks status post wedge labiaplasty.

Once patients have discovered labiaplasty or vaginoplasty as potential solutions to their genital concerns it is only logical that they would approach their gynecologist with questions. Unfortunately, they are told such procedures are unnecessary, potentially dangerous, and to just "live with it." Gynecologists know through experience that variability in size and shape of the labia minora and vulva is physiologically normal; they are not accustomed to navigating aesthetic vulvar concerns but rather medical issues such as dyspareunia, urinary problems such as spraying, stress or urge incontinence, or vaginal itching or discharge. Along with an underappreciation for aesthetic genital concerns, American College of Obstetricians and Gynecologists has condemned any surgical procedures to reduce the labia minora or enhance sexual function in women unless medically indicated.[2,3]

Labiaplasty has been shown to be safe and effective when performed by properly trained individuals.[4] However, despite condemnation by the governing body of gynecologists, many surgeons choose to perform labiaplasty without proper training resulting in complications. Several revision labiaplasty consultations present each year from young teenage girls who have undergone an aggressive trim labiaplasty at a local children's hospital by a gynecologist or plastic surgeon. The deceivingly simple procedure is typically done under insurance, and the outcome is not acceptable to the patient or the parent. Most commonly the labia minora has been overresected

or a large clitoral hood has been left unaddressed by an inexperienced surgeon. The patient and parent are distraught and are either referred to a specialist or seek help online. Visibility on the Internet for terms such as "revision labiaplasty" or "redo labiaplasty" helps direct such inquiries to one's Web site. Treatment options for these patients are often limited, and even the most experienced labiaplasty surgeons struggle to repair the problems.

Staff Education on Procedures

Office staff that interact with patients should be well versed in genital procedures and comfortable discussing genital anatomy with potential patients. The process begins with the initial phone inquiry in which patients may be embarrassed to request a labiaplasty or a vaginal tightening consultation. It is not unusual for patients to be so intimidated that they book a consultation for a more conventional procedure like breast augmentation or abdominoplasty, yet on the day of the consultation reveal they are interested in a labiaplasty. Experienced staff should be able to make patients comfortable on the phone and in person regarding their genital inquiries.

Phone staff as well as physician extenders need to be familiar with the anatomy and comfortable speaking with patients about the topic. It is well worth the surgeon's time to review the anatomy, symptoms, and procedure types with staff and physician extenders. Most patients are interested

Below are a number of statements that women might make about their genitals. Please read each statement, and underline to what extent, if any, this statement applies to you.
A diagram is provided to show the anatomy of the female genitalia.

1. I feel that my genitals are normal in appearance.

Never   Sometimes   Often   Always

2. I feel my genitals are unattractive in appearance

Never   Sometimes   Often   Always

3. I feel my labia are too large

Never   Sometimes   Often   Always

4. I am satisfied with the appearance of my genitals

Never   Sometimes   Often   Always

5. I experience irritation to my labia when exercising/walking

Never   Sometimes   Often   Always

6. I feel, or have felt, conscious in sexual situations because of the appearance of my genitals

Never   Sometimes   Often   Always

7. Embarrassment about the appearance of my genitals spoils my enjoyment of sex

Never   Sometimes   Often   Always

8. I feel discomfort around my genitals when I wear tight clothes

Never   Sometimes   Often   Always

9. I feel that my genital area is visible under tight clothes

Never   Sometimes   Often   Always

10. I worry about the appearance of my vaginal area

Never   Sometimes   Often   Always

11. I feel that my genital area looks asymmetric , or 'lopsided'

Never   Sometimes   Often   Always

Fig. 2. Genital appearance satisfaction scale. (*From* Bramwell R and Morland C. Genital appearance satisfaction in women: the development of a questionnaire and exploration of correlates, Journal of Reproductive and Infant Psychology, 27:1, 15-27, 2009.)

in a labiaplasty, vaginal tightening (vaginoplasty) on nonsurgical vaginal rejuvenation. The consultation coordinator needs to be patient and understand the stress patients feel with verbalizing these embarrassing issues.

Questionnaires

Once patients have booked a consultation, validated questionnaires about sexual function, genital self-image, and urinary symptoms are e-mailed to patients via a secure portal. These surveys help tease out the patient's desires and symptoms before the consultation. Knowledge of sexual dysfunction and genital self-image helps the surgeon understand the motivating factors behind seeking surgery.

The genital appearance satisfaction scale[5,6] (Fig. 2) is an 11-question survey validated for use in women seeking labiaplasty. Answers summarize the patient's perception of their labia regarding size, appearance, and influence on

COPS –L for women seeking labiaplasty

*This questionnaire is about the way you feel about the appearance of your genitalia. The outer lips of your gentialia are called the "labia" Please answer how you feel for **over the past week**.*

Name _____ Date _____

1) How abnormal do you feel your labia is to a sexual partner (if you do **not try to hide your genitalia**) and you do not highlight it to him/her?

```
0        1        2        3        4        5        6        7        8
|_____|_____|_____|_____|_____|_____|_____|_____|
Not at all        Slightly          Moderately        Markedly          Very
abnormal          abnormal          abnormal          abnormal          abnormal
```

2) To what extent do you feel the appearance of your labia are **currently** ugly, unattractive or 'not right'?

```
0        1        2        3        4        5        6        7        8
|_____|_____|_____|_____|_____|_____|_____|_____|
Very              Markedly          Moderately        Slightly          Not at all
ugly or           unattractive      unattractive      unattractive      unattractive
'not right'
```

3) To what extent do your labia **currently** cause you distress?

```
0        1        2        3        4        5        6        7        8
|_____|_____|_____|_____|_____|_____|_____|_____|
Not at all        Slightly          Moderately        Markedly          Extremely
distressing       distressing       distressing       distressing       distressing
```

4) To what extent does thinking about the appearance of your labia **currently** preoccupy you? That is, you think about it a lot and it is hard to stop thinking about it?

```
0        1        2        3        4        5        6        7        8
|_____|_____|_____|_____|_____|_____|_____|_____|
Not at all        Slightly          Moderately        Very              Extremely
preoccupied       preoccupied       preoccupied       preoccupied       preoccupied
```

5) If you **have a regular partner**, to what extent do your concerns about your labia **currently** have an effect on your relationship with an existing partner? (e.g. affectionate feelings, number of arguments, enjoying activities together? **If you do not have a regular partner**, to what extent do your concerns about your labia **currently** have an effect on dating or developing a relationship? (do not include any sexual relationship as this is discussed below).

```
0        1        2        3        4        5        6        7        8
|_____|_____|_____|_____|_____|_____|_____|_____|
Not at all        Slightly          Moderately        Markedly          Extremely
```

Fig. 3. (*A, B*) Cosmetic procedure screening scale for labiaplasty. (*From* Veale D, Eshkevari E, Ellison N, Cardozo L, Robinson D, Kavouni A. Validation of genital appearance satisfaction scale and the cosmetic procedure screening scale for women seeking labiaplasty. *J Psychosom Obstet Gynaecol.* 2013;34(1):46-52.)

sexual function. Understanding the motivation for labiaplasty helps define the aesthetic goals of the patients. Matching these goals with outcomes is important.

The Cosmetic Procedure Screening Questionnaire for Labiaplasty (COPS L) (**Fig. 3**) is a validated 9-question survey used to determine if body dysmorphic disorder (BDD) is present in patients seeking labiaplasty.[7] Preoccupation with genital appearance is a rare presentation of BDD; however, if responses to the COPS L indicate the potential for this disorder, further investigation into the situation is warranted. Proceeding with any surgical intervention on a patient with BDD is fraught with complications as expectations are rarely met. Even though the surgery may be a success, the patient will not be happy.

The Pelvic Organ/Urinary Incontinence Sexual Function Questionnaire (PISQ 12) (**Fig. 4**) is a validated symptom-specific quality-of-life

6) If you **have a regular partner**, to what extent do your concerns about your labia **currently** have an effect on an existing sexual relationship? (e.g. enjoyment of sex, frequency of sexual activity, labia getting trapped in your vagina, only having sex in the dark). **If you do not have a regular partner**, to what extent do your concerns about your labia **currently** stop you from developing a sexual relationship?

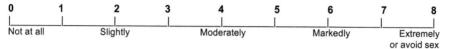

| 0 | 1 | 2 | 3 | 4 | 5 | 6 | 7 | 8 |
| Not at all | | Slightly | | Moderately | | Markedly | | Extremely or avoid sex |

7) To what extent do your concerns about your labia currently interfere with your leisure activities that might involve someone noticing your labia? (e.g., those that might involve public changing rooms or wearing swimsuits)

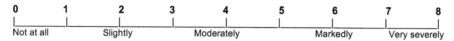

| 0 | 1 | 2 | 3 | 4 | 5 | 6 | 7 | 8 |
| Not at all | | Slightly | | Moderately | | Markedly | | Very severely |

8) How noticeable do you think your labia are in public situations (e.g., in a changing room naked) **if you do not try to deliberately hide your genitalia?**

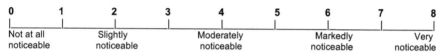

| 0 | 1 | 2 | 3 | 4 | 5 | 6 | 7 | 8 |
| Not at all noticeable | | Slightly noticeable | | Moderately noticeable | | Markedly noticeable | | Very noticeable |

9) How do think the appearance of your labia compare to other women of the same age and ethnic group?

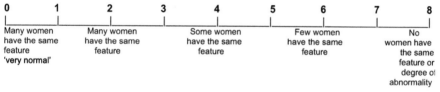

| 0 | 1 | 2 | 3 | 4 | 5 | 6 | 7 | 8 |
| Many women have the same feature 'very normal' | | Many women have the same feature | | Some women have the same feature | | Few women have the same feature | | No women have the same feature or degree of abnormality |

Fig. 3. (*continued*)

questionnaire that assesses sexual function in women with urinary incontinence and/or pelvic floor prolapse.[8] More than 50% of postmenopausal women suffer from some form of stress, urge, or mixed urinary incontinence.[9] Many women seeking surgical and nonsurgical options for improving vaginal laxity suffer from stress urinary incontinence due to anterior vaginal wall laxity or cystocele. Patients with symptomatic organ prolapse (grade 2 or 3) have been found to suffer from sexual dysfunction[10] and require referral to a pelvic floor specialist (urogynecologist).

The Female Sexual Function Index (FSFI) (**Fig. 5**) questionnaire combines inquiries related to sexual function such as pain with intercourse, lubrication issues, desire, and orgasm. Vaginal laxity is usually perceived as a decrease in sensation with intercourse and occurs, although underreported, in up to 80% of women.[11] Vaginal wall laxity, damage to the perineal body, prolapse, and neurovascular injury pertaining to pregnancy and childbirth contribute to the decrease in sensation in some

women. Retrospective studies show that women who undergo vaginal tightening surgery and perineoplasty report improved sexual function.[12]

The Consultation: Defining the Problem

The results of the questionnaires should be reviewed by the physician before entering the consultation room. A preferably female physician extender first gathers vital signs and reviews the pertinent medical history and medications with the patient fully clothed in the examination room. In younger patients who present with a parent, tact must be used in obtaining a sexual history. Patients are frequently embarrassed and uncomfortable discussing their genitalia. Efforts should be taken to discuss the topic in an up-front and matter-of-fact way. The use of anatomic models and diagrams helps alleviate anxiety during the consultation process.

The physician then enters the room with the assistant and begins the conversation with the

Pelvic Organ Prolapse/Urinary Incontinence Sexual Function Questionnaire (PISQ-12)

Instructions: Following are a list of questions about you and your partner's sex life. All information is strictly confidential. Your confidential answers will be used only to help doctors understand what is important to patients about their sex lives. Please check the box that best answers the question for you. While answering the questions, consider your sexuality over the past six months. Thank you for your help.

1. How frequently do you feel sexual desire? This feeling may include wanting to have sex, planning to have sex, feeling frustrated due to lack of sex, etc.

   ☐ Always ☐ Usually ☐ Sometimes ☐ Seldom ☐ Never

2. Do you climax (have an orgasm) when having sexual intercourse with your partner?

   ☐ Always ☐ Usually ☐ Sometimes ☐ Seldom ☐ Never

3. Do you feel sexually excited (turned on) when having sexual activity with your partner?

   ☐ Always ☐ Usually ☐ Sometimes ☐ Seldom ☐ Never

4. How satisfied are you with the variety of sexual activities in you current sex life?

   ☐ Always ☐ Usually ☐ Sometimes ☐ Seldom ☐ Never

5. Do you feel pain during sexual intercourse?

   ☐ Always ☐ Usually ☐ Sometimes ☐ Seldom ☐ Never

6. Are you incontinent of urine (leak urine) with sexual activity?

   ☐ Always ☐ Usually ☐ Sometimes ☐ Seldom ☐ Never

7. Does fear of incontinence (either stool or urine) restrict your sexual activity?

   ☐ Always ☐ Usually ☐ Sometimes ☐ Seldom ☐ Never

8. Do you avoid sexual intercourse because of bulging in the vagina (either the bladder, rectum or vagina falling out?)?

   ☐ Always ☐ Usually ☐ Sometimes ☐ Seldom ☐ Never

9. When you have sex with your partner, do you have negative emotional reactions such as fear, disgust, shame or guilt?

   ☐ Always ☐ Usually ☐ Sometimes ☐ Seldom ☐ Never

10. Does your partner have a problem with erections that affects your sexual activity?

   ☐ Always ☐ Usually ☐ Sometimes ☐ Seldom ☐ Never

11. Does your partner have a problem with premature ejaculation that affects your sexual activity?

   ☐ Always ☐ Usually ☐ Sometimes ☐ Seldom ☐ Never

12. Compared to orgasms you have had in the past, how intense are the orgasms you have had in the past six months?

   ☐ Much less intense ☐ Less intense ☐ Same intensity ☐ More intense ☐ Much more intense

Scoring:

Scores are calculated by totaling the scores for each question with 0=never, 4=always. Reverse scoring is used for items 1,2,3 and 4. The short form questionnaire can be used with up to two missing responses. To handle missing values the sum is calculated by multiplying the number of items by the mean of the answered items. If there are more than two missing responses, the short form no longer accurately predicts long form scores. Short form scores can only be reported as total or on an item basis. Although the short form reflects the content of the three factors in the long form, it is not possible to analyze data at the factor level. To compare long and short form scores multiply the short form score by 2.58 (12/31).

Fig. 4. Pelvic organ prolapse/urinary incontinence sexual questionnaire. (*From* Trang, H., Cuong, P. and Tuyet, H. (2019) Prevalence of Female Sexual Dysfunction among Women with Pelvic Organ Prolapse Diagnosed by Pisq-12 and Related Factors in Hung Vuong Hospital, Vietnam. Open Journal of Obstetrics and Gynecology, 9, 1005-1018.)

patient by thanking the patient for filling out the series of questionnaires and explains that the answers help define the issue at hand. Patients are comforted when they learn that they are not the only ones presenting with complaints of labia minora excess or decreased sexual sensation after having kids. Patients with labia minora excess usually describe a long-standing concern with the appearance of their genitalia. Questions regarding the onset (adolescence, childbirth) of these observations help to create a safe environment to discuss the sensitive issue. It is not uncommon for patients to reveal that a partner commented on the size or shape of their labia minora or laxity of their vagina.

Digital diagrams and photographs are helpful in explaining the vulvar anatomy. It is not uncommon for patients to confuse the labia minora and the

APPENDIX A

Female Sexual Function Index (FSFI)

Subject Identifier _____ Age _____ Date _____

INSTRUCTIONS: These questions ask about your sexual feelings and responses during the past 4 weeks. Please answer the following questions as honestly and clearly as possible. Your responses will be kept completely confidential. In answering these questions the following definitions apply:

Sexual activity can include caressing, foreplay, masturbation and vaginal intercourse.

Sexual intercourse is defined as penile penetration (entry) of the vagina.

Sexual stimulation includes situations like foreplay with a partner, self-stimulation (masturbation), or sexual fantasy.

CHECK ONLY ONE BOX PER QUESTION.

Sexual desire or interest is a feeling that includes wanting to have a sexual experience, feeling receptive to a partner's sexual initiation, and thinking or fantasizing about having sex.

1. Over the past 4 weeks, how **often** did you feel sexual desire or interest?
- Almost always or always
- Most times (more than half the time)
- Sometimes (about half the time)
- A few times (less than half the time)
- Almost never or never

2. Over the past 4 weeks, how would you rate your **level** (degree) of sexual desire or interest?
- Very high
- High
- Moderate
- Low
- Very low or none at all

Sexual arousal is a feeling that includes both physical and mental aspects of sexual excitement. It may include feelings of warmth or tingling in the genitals, lubrication (wetness), or muscle contractions.

3. Over the past 4 weeks, how often did you feel sexually aroused ("turned on") during sexual activity or intercourse?
- No sexual activity
- Almost always or always
- Most times (more than half the time)
- Sometimes (about half the time)
- A few times (less than half the time)
- Almost never or never

4. Over the past 4 weeks, how would you rate your level of sexual arousal ("turn on") during sexual activity or intercourse?
- No sexual activity
- Very high
- High
- Moderate
- Low
- Very low or none at all

5. Over the past 4 weeks, how **confident** were you about becoming sexually aroused during sexual activity or intercourse?
- No sexual activity
- Very high confidence
- High confidence
- Moderate confidence
- Low confidence
- Very low or no confidence

6. Over the past 4 weeks, how **often** have you been satisfied with your arousal (excitement) during sexual activity or intercourse?
- No sexual activity
- Almost always or always
- Most times (more than half the time)
- Sometimes (about half the time)
- A few times (less than half the time)
- Almost never or never

7. Over the past 4 weeks, how **often** did you become lubricated ("wet") during sexual activity or intercourse?
- No sexual activity
- Almost always or always
- Most times (more than half the time)
- Sometimes (about half the time)
- A few times (less than half the time)
- Almost never or never

8. Over the past 4 weeks, how **difficult** was it to become lubricated ("wet") during sexual activity or intercourse?
- No sexual activity
- Extremely difficult or impossible
- Very difficult
- Difficult
- Slightly difficult
- Not difficult

9. Over the past 4 weeks, how often did you **maintain** your lubrication ("wetness") until completion of sexual activity or intercourse?
- No sexual activity
- Almost always or always
- Most times (more than half the time)
- Sometimes (about half the time)
- A few times (less than half the time)
- Almost never or never

10. Over the past 4 weeks, how **difficult** was it to maintain your lubrication ("wetness") until completion of sexual activity or intercourse?
- No sexual activity
- Extremely difficult or impossible
- Very difficult
- Difficult
- Slightly difficult
- Not difficult

Fig. 5. Female sexual satisfaction scale. (*Adapted from* Rosen R, Brown C, Heiman J, et al. The Female Sexual Function Index (FSFI): a multidimensional self-report instrument for the assessment of female sexual function. *J Sex Marital Ther.* 2000;26(2):191-208.)

labia majora. Most are bothered by enlarged labia minora protruding beyond the labia majora in the standing position.[13] However, perimenopausal women may have concerns about the aged appearance of a long vulvar cleft (standing view) due to long lax labia majora. The tremendous variation in normal anatomy of the region should be emphasized.

Once the patient is familiar with the anatomy, the surgical options can be shown. Labia minora reduction procedures such as the wedge or edge trim are easily demonstrated with diagrams or animations during the consultation. Patients appreciate the demonstration of the different procedures as well as the location of the scars. Some patients will try to dictate the type of technique they prefer based on their "research" on the Internet. The surgeon should gracefully respond that outcomes are optimized when the surgeon's experience and skill are used to dictate the technique.

The scar for labia majora excision is more visible and much longer that the average labia minora reduction scar. It is important to show patients a diagram of where the scar will be located between the labia minora and the labia majora. In addition, it behooves the surgeon to explain the relationship of the labia minora size and length to the labia majora. Patients need to understand that reduction of the labia majora can increase the relative protrusion of the labia minora.

Older perimenopausal patients frequently have labia majora complaints. These patients dislike the skin laxity in lithotomy position and the elongated vulvar cleft in the standing position. Labia majora frequently increases in size with pregnancy due to weight gain, varicose vein engorgement, and round ligament stretch. These are difficult problems to address once the labia majora is deflated because skin quality worsens with age (estrogen starved) and the fibroseptal network that anchors the labia majora skin to the inferior pubic ramus has been stretched out.

Patients may request clitoral hood reduction in hopes of increasing sexual sensation and the ability to achieve a clitoral orgasm. Intuitively it seems that less tissue surrounding the clitoral glans would allow for easier stimulation. Patients should be warned that surgical debulking of the clitoral hood may not result in increased sensation of the clitoris. The surgeon should explain that 2 to 3 mm of hooding over the clitoris in the flaccid state is normal to prevent glans exposure and chronic discomfort.

The review of before and after photographs helps define the patient's vision of their vulva postoperatively. Patients can be asked to give their opinion on a variety of results. Photographs should be in the standing and lithotomy positions. Young patients in their 20s tend to desire a very trim appearance of the vulva with minimal labia minora show, whereas older patients may consider such results are unnatural. The review also serves as a test of the patient's scar tolerance and appreciation of postoperative asymmetry. If the patient cannot identify a pleasing result or is hypercritical of the results, thought must be given to perhaps not proceeding with surgery.

Detailed Gynecologic History

Patients should be asked as part of their intake forms several detailed questions regarding their gynecologic history. Young patients may have never seen a gynecologist because many are not sexually active at the time that they seek labiaplasty. It is a good practice in sexually active patients to document a negative Papanicolaou test within the past few years. Questions regarding sexual activity are important so staff as well as the physician should be comfortable soliciting a good sexual history.

The parity status of patients as well as the type of delivery and history of tearing or episiotomy are important especially in the vaginal laxity patient. Dyspareunia whether from infolding of the labia minora or an irritated episiotomy scar is important to document preoperatively. Patients should be counseled that neither labiaplasty nor vaginoplasty is a solution for dyspareunia of unknown cause. Pain and severe vulvar itching in women older than 50 years may be due to vulvar lichen sclerosis[14] and should be referred to a dermatologist or gynecologist for treatment.

Enlarged labia minora and/or clitoral hood may divert the urinary stream and cause spraying. This mechanical obstruction may be improved with labiaplasty and/or clitoral hood reduction. However, urinary spraying in perimenopausal women may be due to urethral synechiae so determining the cause of the stream divergence is important. Patients with recurrent urinary tract infections and yeast infections should be warned of the potential perioperative need for treatment. Bacterial vaginosis is frequently encountered during the perioperative period, and treatment with topical intravaginal metronidazole gel may be necessary.

Physical Examination

Patients interested in vulvar aesthetic procedures should be examined in both the standing and lithotomy positions. An examination table with stirrups is helpful in that the entire perineum and vulva can be visualized. The mons height and degree of laxity should be documented. It is not uncommon for postpartum women to have a degree of mons ptosis that affects the appearance of the labia majora; this may be demonstrated to patients by giving them a handheld mirror and showing them the effect of mons elevation on the appearance of the labia majora.

The labia majora are then evaluated for subcutaneous thickness and skin laxity. It is useful to note the presence of significant mobility of the interlabial groove between the majora and the labia minora. If there is significant lateral distraction of the labia minora with lateral tension of the majora one must be wary of aggressive majora reduction. According to Hunter,[15] up to 50% of the horizontal width of the labia majora may be safely resected; however, this may result in splaying open of the labia minora. Ideally, the posterior portion of the labia majora should curve inward toward the posterior fourchette. In a postpartum patient with a gaping introitus the posterior majora will be separated apart; this will only be improved with a perineoplasty not a labia majora reduction alone.

The labia minora size, symmetry, shape, and edge thickness is then noted. Asymmetry is very common and should be pointed out to the patient. The presence of a double fold or anterior labial fold may affect the choice of surgical resection. Wedge resections are best performed posterior to the junction of the clitoral frenulum and the anterior labial fold.[16] Large redundant labia minora with a wide arc may require 2 wedge resections per side to avoid narrowing of the introitus.[17] Finally, the posterior fourchette should be assessed. Some labia minora are connected posteriorly, which may influence the choice of labiaplasty technique.

The clitoral hood is then assessed for length, width, and thickness. Particular attention should be paid to the length of the clitoral frenula and amount of clitoral glans show. The clitoris itself should then be gently palpated by compressing the clitoral hood after notifying the patient of the intention. Clitoromegaly either primary or secondary may be the source of hood protrusion. If the clitoris is enlarged, referral to a specialist for genetic counseling or a urologist for clitoral reduction[18] should be discussed with the patient.

The introitus itself is then evaluated. The visibility of hymenal remnants, the effacement of the mucosa, and the width of the introitus help determine if perineoplasty may be warranted. Patients may not be aware that a reduction of the labia minora may expose a widened introitus. Their focus is only on the enlarged labia not what is below them. Next the patient is asked to bare down or Valsalva. A posterior bulge may suggest a rectocele and an anterior bulge a cystocele. Symptomatic prolapse may warrant referral to a urogynecologist for evaluation and treatment.

If the patient reports a decrease in sensation with intercourse and vaginal laxity, the vagina should be assessed. First the color and condition of the mucosa should be documented. Evidence of excoriation, unstable episiotomy scars or thinning of the tissues will affect the type of procedure and/or treatment performed. For example, menopausal patients usually have loss of rugae and pallor of the mucosa, which may benefit from topical estrogen therapy in the perioperative period.

Patients frequently report that they have complained to their gynecologists about vaginal laxity and decreased sensation with intercourse but were told it is a normal consequence of pregnancy and aging. If symptoms and signs of significant prolapse are not present patients are encouraged to do Kegel exercises or are referred for pelvic floor physical therapy. Studies have shown an improvement in postmenopausal sexual function with pelvic floor muscular training.[19]

To assess vaginal laxity on physical examination the back wall of the vagina should be palpated in the lithotomy position for any posterior floor weakness. Patients are asked to perform a Kegel[20] maneuver while the posterior wall of the vagina is palpated with the index finger in about 2 cm. The strength of the pelvic floor contracture may be quantified with the modified Oxford scale (**Table 1**).[21] Then the patient is asked to perform a Valsalva maneuver while visualizing the introitus with the labia minora separated. Bulging of either the anterior wall (cystocele) or posterior wall (rectocele) should be noted.

RECOMMENDATIONS

Once the examination is completed, the surgical plan is formulated. It is not uncommon for more than one procedure to be performed at the same time. Patients may not understand what is contributing to the "saggy" or "old" appearance of their vulva. In younger patients, labia minora asymmetry or enlargement is the chief complaint. Older patients who have had children or significant weight shifts are frequently concerned with the overall vulvar appearance and labia majora laxity.

Table 1 Modified Oxford scale by Laycock	
Oxford Grading Scale by Laycock	
0	No muscle activity
1	Minor muscle "flicker"
2	Weak muscle activity without a circular contraction
3	Moderate muscle contraction
4	Good muscle contraction
5	Strong muscle contraction

From Fitz FF, Stüpp L, Costa TF, Sartori MG, Girão MJ, Castro RA. Correlation between maximum voluntary contraction and endurance measured by digital palpation and manometry: An observational study. Rev Assoc Med Bras (1992). 2016;62(7):635-640.

Defining the problem areas is important to be able to meet patients' expectations.

A gaping introitus in a multiparous patient (Fig. 6) may be more apparent after a labiaplasty. The surgeon needs to do a complete vulvar assessment and show the patient what will be unveiled if a labiaplasty alone is performed. Most patients are well educated via the Internet on options for vulvar aesthetic and functional surgery. They not only want to look good and feel confident but also want to improve their sexual function. Some studies show that perineoplasty improves sexual function for both the man and the woman.[22] There is a dearth of clinical outcomes studies on surgical procedures done to enhance women's sexual function. This is by far a contrast with the amount of literature currently available on procedures and products to enhance male sexual function.

Once the procedure has been determined, informed consent is discussed. As with other plastic surgical procedures, scars will be visible and may become thickened, although this is rare along the labia minora and clitoral hood. Wound dehiscence is the most common complication of wedge labiaplasty.[4] Scar visibility and hypertrophy is more common with labia majora reductions than minora reductions. Splaying of the labia minora and widening of the introitus in the coronal plane is another complication of labia majora reduction.

Perineoplasty and vaginoplasty may result albeit rarely in permanent dyspareunia and visible scar deformity. The importance of documenting preoperative dyspareunia cannot be emphasized enough. In patients with vaginal laxity and a thinned posterior vaginal wall, a rectovaginal fistula is a known risk of vaginoplasty and should be discussed with patients preoperatively. Women interested in vaginal tightening procedures often seek to achieve orgasm during intercourse without direct clitoral glans stimulation. Most women are unable to achieve orgasm during intercourse by penile penetration alone, and patients hoping to reach this goal should be told it is possible but highly unlikely to occur after vaginoplasty and/or perineoplasty.

In conclusion, the female aesthetic consultation requires time and patience on the part of the office staff and surgeon. Patients are usually anxious and frequently have waited years to gather the courage to seek out a consultation for elective genital surgery due to the shroud of guilt associated with these procedures. Patients deserve to be educated on vulvar anatomy, its variations as well as aberrancies, and safe and effective treatment options. Surgeons need to seek appropriate training to perform elective genital procedures, which unfortunately is inadequate in most plastic surgery and nearly all gynecology residencies. These obstacles need to be tackled to have a safe and successful aesthetic female genital practice.

CLINICS CARE POINTS

- Clinical staff should be well versed in genital aesthetic procedures and be comfortable in discussing the topic with patients.
- Validated questionnaires regarding sexual function should be distributed to patients before the consultation because they help define the motivations for seeking genital procedures as well as any preexisting pathologic condition.
- Digital diagrams of vulvar anatomy during the consultation help patients understand anatomy and the areas that may benefit from surgical or nonsurgical treatment.
- Before and after photographs should be shown to patients to educate them on scar location and postoperative asymmetry. The reaction of patients to average results is important because unrealistic expectations may be unveiled.

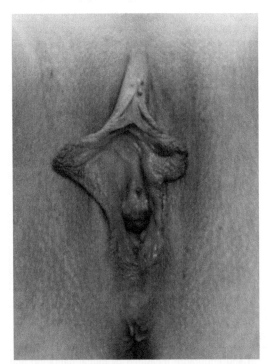

Fig. 6. A 28-year-old female with labia minora asymmetry and a widened introitus.

- A proctor should be present for the consultation and physical examination. A handheld mirror given to the patient helps with identifying anatomic variations that may impact surgical outcome.

DISCLOSURE

Book royalties from Thieme for my textbook *Female Cosmetic Genital Surgery: Concepts, Classification and Techniques*, 2017. IBSN-13: 978 to 1,626,236,493. Paid speaker InMode. No payments received since 2018. No conflicts.

REFERENCES

1. Statistics, surveys and trends. The aesthetic society unveils 2022 plastic surgery predictions from board-certified plastic surgeons. Available at: https://www.surgery.org/media/news-releases/americans-spent-over-87-billion-on-aesthetic-plastic-surgery-in-the-first-6-months-of-2021-. Accessed March 20, 2022.

2. Hamori CA. Teen labiaplasty: a response to the May 2016 American College of Obstetricians and gynecologists (ACOG) recommendations on labiaplasty in adolescents. Aesthet Surg J 2016;36(Issue 7): 807–9.

3. FAQs on vaginal rejuvenation, vaginoplasty and other cosmetic genital surgery. Committee on Gynecologic Practice. (ACOG committee opinion Number 795) Elective Female Genital Cosmetic Surgery. Vol. 135, No. 1. 2020. Available at: https://www.acog.org/clinical/clinical-guidance/committee-opinion/articles/2020/01/elective-female-genital-cosmetic-surgery.

4. Bucknor A, Chen AD, Egeler S, et al. Indications and predictors of postoperative sequelae in 451 consecutive cases. Aesthet Surg J 2018;38(6):644–53.

5. Veale D, Eshkevari E, Ellison N, et al. Validation of genital appearance satisfaction scale and the cosmetic procedure screening scale for women seeking labiaplasty. J Psychosom Obstet Gynaecol 2013;34(1):46–52.

6. Bramwell Ros, Morland Claire. Genital appearance satisfaction in women: the development of a questionnaire and exploration of correlates. J Reprod Infant Psychol 2009;27(1):15–27.

7. Veale David, Ellison Nell, Werner Tom, et al. Development of a cosmetic procedure screening questionnaire (COPS) for body dysmorphic disorder. J Plast Reconstr Aesthet Surg JPRAS 2012;65: 530–2.

8. Rogers RG, Coates KW, Kammerer-Doak D, et al. A short form of the pelvic organ prolapse/urinary incontinence sexual questionnaire (PISQ-12). Int Urogynecol J Pelvic Floor Dysfunct 2003;14(3):164–8.

9. Kołodyńska G, Zalewski M, Rożek-Piechura K. Urinary incontinence in postmenopausal women - causes, symptoms, treatment. Prz Menopauzalny 2019;18(1):46–50.

10. Polland Allison, Duong Vi, Furuya Rachel, et al. Description of vaginal laxity and prolapse and correlation with sexual function (DeVeLoPS). Sex Med 2021;9:100443.

11. Campbell P, Krychman M, Gray T, et al. Self-reported vaginal laxity—Prevalence, impact, and associated symptoms in women attending a urogynecology clinic. J Sex Med 2018;15:1515–7.

12. Goodman MP, Placik OJ, Benson RH 3rd, et al. A large multicenter outcome study of female genital plastic surgery. J Sex Med 2010;7(4 Pt 1):1565–77. Epub 2009 Nov 12. PMID: 19912495.

13. Hamori CA. Postoperative clitoral hood deformity after labiaplasty. Aesthet Surg J 2013;33(Issue 7): 1030–6.

14. Corazza M, Schettini N, Zedde P, et al. Vulvar lichen sclerosus from pathophysiology to therapeutic approaches: evidence and prospects. Biomedicines 2021;9(8):950. Published 2021 Aug 3.

15. Hunter JG. Labia minora, labia majora, and clitoral hood alteration: experience-based recommendations. Aesthet Surg J 2016;36(Issue 1):71–9.

16. Hamori C, Banwell P and Alinsod R. Female Cosmetic Genital Surgery: Concepts, Classification and Techniques. Published 2017.

17. Alter GJ. Aesthetic labia minora and clitoral hood reduction using extended central wedge resection. Plast Reconstr Surg 2008;122(6):1780–9.

18. Rawat J, Singh S. Sensation-preserving clitoral reduction surgery: a preliminary report of our experience. Afr J Paediatr Surg 2022;19(1):23–6.

19. Franco MM, et al. Pelvic floor muscle training effect in sexual function in postmenopausal women: a randomized controlled trial. J Sex Med 2021;18(7): 1236–44.

20. Kegel A. Progressive resistance exercise in the functional restoration of the perineal muscles. Am J Obstet Gynecol 1948;56:238–48.

21. Laycock J. Clinical evaluation of the pelvic floor. In: Pelvic floor re-education, principles and practice. New York, NY: Springer; 1994. p. 42.

22. Ulubay M, Keskin U, Fidan U, et al. Safety, efficiency, and outcomes of perineoplasty: treatment of the sensation of a wide vagina. Biomed Res Int 2016; 2016:2495105.

Labia Minora Reduction Using Central Wedge Technique: Central Wedge Technique

Gary J. Alter, MD*

KEYWORDS

• Labia minora reduction • Labiaplasty • Clitoral hood reduction • Female genital aesthetic surgery

KEY POINTS

- The central wedge labiaplasty preserves normal labial anatomy.
- A four-layer closure with 5-0 Monocryl on a TF needle minimizes separations and perforations.
- The introitus must be wide enough to fit two fingerbreadths.
- Asymmetry of the labia can be corrected in most cases using multiple techniques.
- There is a high patient satisfaction.

In recent decades, especially in the last 10 years, women and men are more aware of genital appearance. Self-esteem is often closely mirrored and dependent on a person's perception of his/her genitalia, both functionally and more recently aesthetically. A woman who views her vulvar area as being unattractive can cause her to socially isolate and be less confident sexually and with interpersonal relationships. As men are now also more closely attuned to genital anatomy, their negative reaction to the appearance of a female partner can be devastating to the woman's ego and confidence.

The onset of the heightened genital awareness can be traced to visual media, both printed and video, along with the fashionable tendency for large numbers of women to remove most or all genital hair. More younger women are now knowledgeable of their anatomy, whereas older women and men often have little knowledge of vulvar anatomy. It is not unusual for an older woman to state that she never looks at her vulvar region but is still self-conscious of its appearance. As styles and sexual openness have changed, the demand for female genital aesthetic surgery has exploded. The aesthetic ideal for the vulva has not been universally accepted as different people have different aesthetic tastes and goals.

The most common female genital aesthetic procedure is a labia minora reduction or labiaplasty. In general, women want the labia minora to be within the labia majora when standing, to be relatively thin, and to be lightly colored. Traditionally, this has been performed by trimming the labia minora edges. All too often, the trimming is done without much concern for a meticulous aesthetic result. Surgeons in the past, and unfortunately many in the present, reduce or remove the labia minora often with casual excision and suturing. This leads to a vast number of women with unsatisfactory or devastating results. If an insecure woman is mangled by an uncaring surgeon, her self-esteem plummets even further, and her faith in doctors is permanently reduced or destroyed.

The central wedge labiaplasty was developed to eliminate the innate disadvantages of most trimming labiaplasties. In this wedge procedure, the area of the greatest protrusion, which usually has the thickest and darkest-colored tissue, is removed with a pie-slice, "V", or wedge excision, and then the resulting edges are sutured together. It, thus, retains the normal labial edge and anatomy with usually no readily visible scars[1] (**Figs. 1** and **2**).

Division of Plastic Surgery, University of California at Los Angeles, 416 North, Bedford Drive, Suite 400, Beverly Hills, CA 90210, USA
* Corresponding author.
E-mail address: altermd@altermd.com

Clin Plastic Surg 49 (2022) 447–453
https://doi.org/10.1016/j.cps.2022.06.002

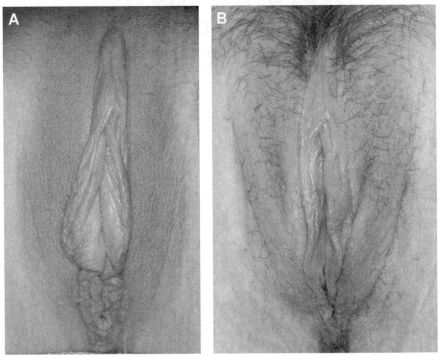

Fig. 1. A 31-year-old woman for routine labiaplasty. (*A*). Pre-operation. (*B*) Post-operation at 3 months.

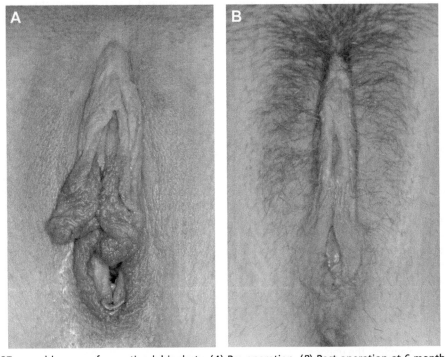

Fig. 2. A 37-year-old woman for routine labiaplasty. (*A*) Pre-operation. (*B*) Post-operation at 6 months.

TECHNIQUE

The patient is placed in the lithotomy position in stirrups in the examination room in consultation. She is given a hand mirror to watch the explanation of the procedure and the proposed outcome.

The surgery is done in the operating room in lithotomy position usually under general anesthesia. Small or unilateral labiaplasties can be done under local anesthesia. However, a routine labiaplasty can take up to a couple of hours, which can be unsettling for many women. Marking of the labia and lateral hood should ideally be done before injecting local anesthesia as the injection can cause swelling and distortion of the tissues. Therefore, general anesthesia improves the accuracy, ease, and comfort of markings as local anesthesia, even with numbing cream, can be uncomfortable and imprecise.

A central wedge or "V" excision is marked in the most protuberant area, which usually includes the thickest and often the darkest area of the labium[1] (**Figs. 1** and **2**; **Figs. 3** and **4**). The upper labial marking is usually at or near the junction of the frenulum and clitoral hood, whereas the lower marking is placed to achieve a straight labium without tension (see **Figs. 3** and **4**).Tension at the suture line will create a tendency for stretching of the scar and increases the possibility of a minor or major dehiscence. Also, care must be taken to assure that the introitus will fit two fingerbreadths, so tightness of the suture line and a high posterior vaginal lip must be assessed. The "V" marking goes internally to end before the hymen and can be angled any direction to achieve an optimal result. The lateral marking extends along the labium and can be curved up along the clitoral hood in an extended hockey stick design to remove any dog-ear or to excise excess lateral clitoral hood skin with subcutaneous tissue (see **Fig. 4**). Do not extend the lateral marking across the labial sulcus as this is deforming. Thus, the external "V" is not a mirror of the internal "V." If needed, the lateral marking can also be curved more medial-laterally to excise hypertrophic or

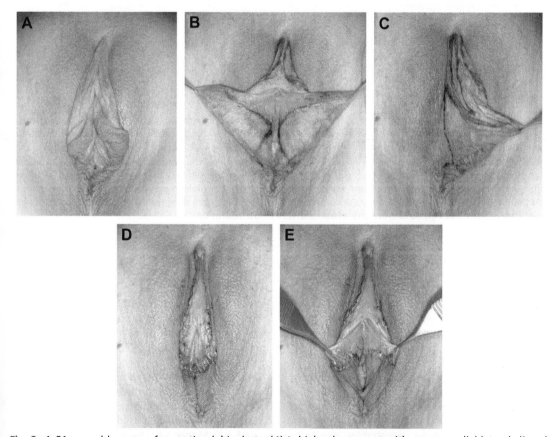

Fig. 3. A 21-year-old woman for routine labiaplasty. (*A*) Labial enlargement with excess medial-lateral clitoral hood skin. (*B*) Labia open. The upper mark for each labium is near the convergence of the frenulum and lateral hood. (*C*) Each central wedge lateral excision ends at the labial sulcus. The hyperkeratotic medial-lateral clitoral hood tissue is excised separately as a vertical ellipse on each side. (*D, E*) Post-operation.

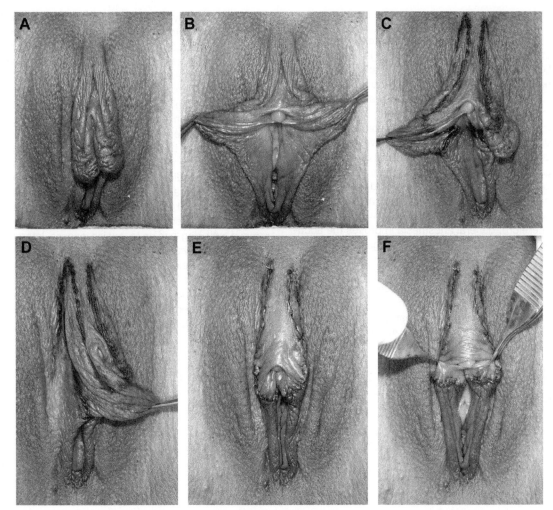

Fig. 4. A 21-year-old woman for routine labiaplasty. (*A, B*) Labial enlargement with long frenula and excess lateral clitoral hood folds. (*C*) Each anterior wedge marking is made where the frenulum appears to blend with the clitoral hood. Adjustments made need to be made if the frenulum is very long. The posterior mark is made where the anterior marking meets without tension. (*D*) Each bilateral lateral hood marking extends as a curved hockey stick design to remove the extra fold. (*E, F*) Post-operation.

highly pigmented medial clitoral hood skin or folds. Alternatively, these medial folds can be removed by ending the wedge at the lateral labium and doing a separate vertical ellipse of the medial hood tissue (see **Fig. 3**). Asymmetry of the hood and labia are common, so the markings are adjusted to correct this as almost all women are concerned about symmetry.

Once the markings are checked, infiltration along the suture lines is performed with 1% xylocaine with epinephrine and $\frac{1}{4}$% marcaine. Only a few ccs are needed along the markings as more infiltration will cause hematomas, swelling, and distortion. Loupe magnification is extremely helpful in performing a meticulous procedure. An incision is made along the medial and lateral

markings just deep enough to go through the skin and mucosa. As much subcutaneous tissue as possible is saved as a strong subcutaneous closure is necessary to prevent dehiscence and perforations. Excess subcutaneous tissue can be removed from the sides of the lateral labium if it is too bulky. Care needs to be taken to prevent clitoral injury.

One side is closed first starting at the labial tip. The only sutures used in the procedure are a 5-0 Monocryl on an atraumatic TF needle. The subcutaneous tissue is closed in two layers of interrupted 5-0 Monocryl. The medial subcutaneous tissue is closed first taking a small amount of tissue then the lateral. After the medial closure, excess subcutaneous tissue is excised laterally before or during the lateral closure. The external leading edge is closed with interrupted vertical mattress 5-0 Monocryl sutures, which are placed medial and lateral. The most medial mucosal closure is done with a running suture. The lateral labial skin is closed with interrupted simple or mattress sutures. The lateral hood is closed with running 5-0 Monocryl in the subcutaneous layer and a subcuticular suture in the skin to avoid cross-hatch scars (see **Fig. 4**). The opposite side is then reduced. Adjustments of the markings of the second labium may need to be done after the closure of the first side.

Asymmetry is not uncommon with labia, so various techniques can be used to resolve it. If only one labium needs to be reduced, the angle of excision can be modified to achieve symmetry (**Fig. 5**). Some women have a long posterior labium, so a second more posterior wedge can be performed on one or both sides. A thicker posterior labium may be present unilaterally or bilaterally. In that case, a vertical lateral and/or medial ellipse along the sides can be performed according a variation reported by Choi[2] (**Fig. 6**). The skin with possibly a little subcutaneous tissue can be excised to make the labia thinner and more symmetric or appealing. The ellipse(s) are closed also with interrupted 5-0 Monocryl.

If the patient has very large, wide, long labia, the medial "V" may extend too far into the introitus and possibly cause overtightening of the introitus. In those cases, a modification of the custom flask

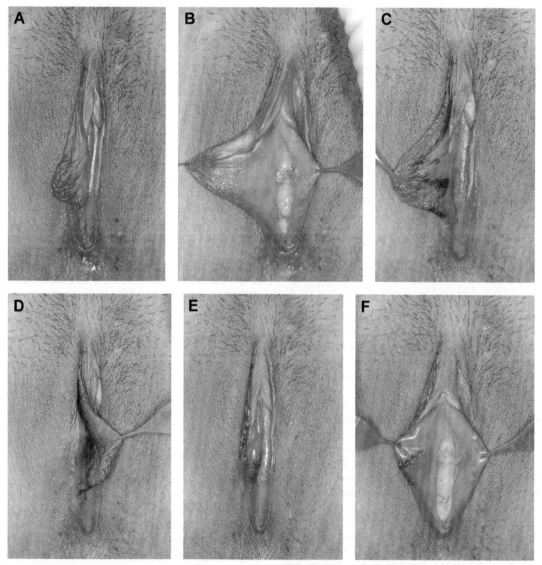

Fig. 5. A 30-year-old woman with right labium minus enlargement. (*A, B*) Pre-operation. (*C*) Medial marking to create symmetry. (*D*) Lateral marking. (*E*) Post-operation. (*F*) Post-operation with labia open.

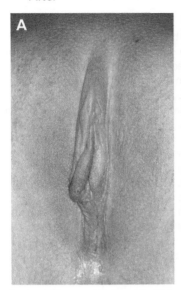 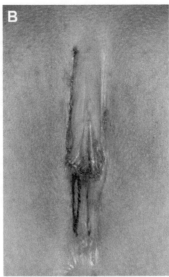 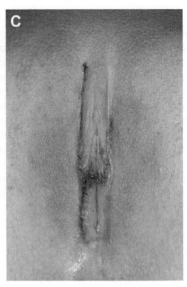

Fig. 6. A 17-year-old girl with thicker right posterior labium. (*A*) Pre-operation. (*B*) Marking for lateral excision. (*C*) Post-operation with symmetry.

labiaplasty medially will prevent this.[3] The anterior and posterior marks on the labial edge are the same. A 1-cm mark is made at right angles to each medial mark, and a back cut of this 1-cm labial width is made along the medial labium anterior and posterior. An incision is made along the junction of the inner labial skin and vaginal mucosa, so the length of both back cuts needs to equal this line resulting in an internal "T" closure. The markings laterally are the same as with a routine labiaplasty. The chance of a minor edge dehiscence is somewhat higher with this technique, but it is easy to do a revision later.

The vaginal introitus must be able to fit two fingerbreadths, so the posterior lip must be evaluated before and during the procedure. If there is a thin upward lip, then this can be cut in the midline and closed horizontally. If there is a high thick posterior lip, this should be noticed before starting the case and adjustments determined in advance. The posterior lip may need to be opened and reconstructed with possible vaginal mucosa advancement to the perineum.

If a perineoplasty or vaginal tightening is performed at the same time as a labiaplasty, then the surgeon should be cognizant of overtightening the posterior introitus. He may want to close external to the hymen after the labiaplasty but this varies depending on the situation. Usually, the perineoplasty is performed before the labiaplasty to set the labiaplasty parameters.

Often, other procedures such as a labia majora reduction, clitoropexy with hood reduction, or clitoris reduction are performed in conjunction with the labiaplasty. Exparel is injected at the end of the procedure.

POST-OPERATION CARE

Keflex is given for 1 day and bacitracin is applied for a day. Ice is applied for 48 hours. Showering with lukewarm water is allowed in 1 day. Gentle washing with a mild soap like Ivory or Dove is allowed in a week. A squirt bottle is used after urinating with gentle dabbing for weeks. Exercise is allowed in 3 to 4 weeks and intercourse in 6 weeks. The sutures dissolve in 3 to 6 weeks and can cause itching, which is partially relieved by Atarax and Dermoplast spray.

RESULTS

If the surgery is meticulously performed according to the method outlined, the complication rate is extremely low.[1] About 5% of the patients will have a minor separation at the tip of the labiaplasty. These usually become unnoticeable or minimally noticeable within 1 to 2 months. If still visible, then a repair under local is easily done at 5 months. Perforations are very uncommon with the four-layer closure, whereas a major dehiscence is very rare and usually only occurs in smokers, with an infection, or due to poor technique. Discomfort lasting over 2 months is also very uncommon. Over 95% of patients are happy or very happy after their labiaplasty.

DISCUSSION

The central wedge labiaplasty was invented to maintain normal anatomy and eliminate the disadvantages of other labiaplasty techniques.

Trimming techniques that eliminate the normal labia edge, whether using a laser, scalpel, scissors, or radiofrequency device have multiple disadvantages including the tendency to over-resect; frequent asymmetry; difficulty making a smooth transition at the junction of the frenulum, upper labium, and clitoral hood; the loss of the normal labial edge that is replaced by a scar-line that can be wide with color contrast, especially in thick labia; occasional separation of the longitudinal suture line with wide scars; the increased tendency for the scar line to have tender, painful areas; the often cross-hatch unsightly scars with scallops; and the release of the frenula and hood that can cause the hood and clitoris to rotate anteriorly and increase introital length.[4] The advantages of the trim are the quicker surgical time and the elimination of dark pigment on some women with thin labia. Nonetheless, most surgeons carefully performing trimming labiaplasties on appropriate patients achieve a high level of patient satisfaction.[5–7]

The Choi technique removes medial and lateral labial sides, which reduces labial protrusion but not the linear longitudinal length of the labia.[2] This can result in redundant, convoluted labia. This technique is useful as an adjunct to the wedge technique when further reduction of protrusion is needed after the wedge is completed.

The posterior wedge technique advances the anterior labia posteriorly, which makes the anterior flap longer with proven less vascularity than the central wedge.[8,9] The reduced vascularity raises the risk of a minor or major dehiscence. It also advances and leaves the thickest and most pigmented portion of the labium posteriorly, which prevents an ideal aesthetic outcome.

The advantages of the central wedge are easier ability to achieve symmetry, the preservation of the normal labial edge, the rare chronic discomfort at the incision lines, less postoperative pain in most instances, and the difficulty to over-resect. The disadvantages are the longer surgical time requiring more surgical skill, the possibility of a color mismatch at the incision line (which usually blends over time), the preservation of the dark labial edge (despite the usual removal of the darkest tissue in the wedge), and the rare dehiscence if performed carefully.

SUMMARY

The central wedge labiaplasty is a major advancement in the surgical treatment to reduce enlarged labia minora. In contrast to the other labiaplasty techniques, this method eliminates the most protuberant portion of the labia minora while maintaining the normal anatomy, labial edge, and sensation with minimal scars and complications. Patients are almost universally happy with their result as long as the procedure is performed meticulously and with keen aesthetic judgment.

CLINICS CARE POINTS

- The central wedge labiaplasty preserves normal labial anatomy.
- A four-layer closure with 5-0 Monocryl on a TF needle minimizes separations and perforations. Do not close under tension.
- Loupe magnification is very helpful.
- The introitus must be wide enough to fit two fingerbreadths. Beware of tightening the vaginal introitus too much when doing vaginal tightening and/or a perineoplasty, or when reducing very wide, long labia.
- Asymmetry of the labia can be corrected in most cases using multiple techniques.
- Smokers have a higher complication rate.

DISCLOSURE

The author has no disclosures.

REFERENCES

1. Alter GJ. Aesthetic labia minora and clitoral hood reduction using extended central wedge resection. Plast Reconstr Surg 2008;122:1780–9.
2. Choi HY, Kim KT. A new method for aesthetic reduction to the labia minora (the deepithelialized reduction labiaplasty). Plast Reconstr Surg 2000;105:419–22.
3. Gonzalez F, Dass D, Almeida B. Custom flask labiaplasty. Ann Plast Surg 2015;75:266–71.
4. Alter GJ. Labia minora reconstruction using clitoral hood flaps, wedge excisions, and YV advancement flaps. Plast Reconstr Surg 2011;127:2356–63.
5. Goodman MP, Placik OJ, Matlock DL, et al. Evaluation of body image and sexual satisfaction in women undergoing female genital plastic/cosmetic surgery. Aesthet Surg J 2016;36(9):1048–57.
6. Lista F, Mistry BD, Singh Y, et al. The safety of aesthetic labiaplasty: a plastic surgery experience. Aesthet Surg J 2015;35(6):689–95.
7. Abbed T, Chen C, Kortesis B, et al. Labiaplasty: current trends of ASAPS members. Aesthet Surg J 2018; 38(8):NP114–7.
8. Munhoz AM, Filassi JR, Ricci MD, et al. Aesthetic labia minora reduction with inferior wedge resection and superior pedicle flap reconstruction. Plast Reconstr Surg 2006;118:1237–47.
9. Georgiou CA, Benatar M, Dumas P, et al. A cadaveric study of the arterial blood supply of the labia minora. Plast Reconstr Surg 2015;136(1):167–78.

Curvilinear Labiaplasty and Clitoral Hood Reduction Surgery

David Ghozland, MD[a], Red Alinsod, MD[b],*

KEYWORDS

- Labiaplasty • Clitoral hood reduction • Radiofrequency • Barbie look • Hybrid look
- Curvilinear labiaplasty • Linear excision labiaplasty

KEY POINTS

- Curvilinear labiaplasty is an effective surgical technique with the fewest risks. It can achieve the appearance the patient desires in almost all cases.
- Labiaplasty is best done in an office setting. Local anesthesia in an awake setting without an intravenous line is exceptionally safe.
- The same basic surgical technique is performed to achieve the degree of labial reduction the patient wants.
- Clitoral hood reduction surgery is often recommended to achieve a balanced and symmetric appearance.
- Radiosurgical tools and techniques are exceptionally precise with minimal lateral heat spread.

CASE STUDY

Erica is an active 36-year-old mother of three children and an athletic trainer. For years, she has felt uncomfortable when wearing her usual workout clothes and aesthetically not pleasing. In her situation, her enlarged labias have caused discomfort and chaffing when rubbing against her clothing. This led to painful intercourse and near-constant irritation bringing her into our office for a surgical consultation. Using a curvilinear approach, we were able to correct the issue with minor recovery time.

A labiaplasty minora surgery and clitoral hood reduction is an outpatient procedure either performed under local or general anesthesia that serves to improve the aesthetic and functional quality of the vulva.[1–3] The procedure not only restores confidence and self-esteem but improves discomfort and irritation for many women. Presently, labiaplasty minora procedures are one of the most frequently performed aesthetic vaginal surgical procedures. Considering normal anatomic variations, Hodgkinson and Hait[4] defined the ideal aesthetic picture of female external genitalia as the one in which the labia minora are small and not larger than the labia majora.

The Technique Used

After years of performing labiaplasty surgery and experimenting with various styles of surgical technique, our preferred approach to performing this procedure is the curved linear technique (sometimes referred to as curvilinear excision, cutting, or amputation techniques) or elliptical excision.[2,4,5] In our opinion it is the most effective with the fewest risks. The incision runs along the length of the labia. It allows the surgeon to remove darker pigmentation often found on the edges of the labia and more accurately create the new shape of the labia as determined by the patient. However, it should be noted that the technique is

[a] 11645 Wilshire Boulevard, Suite 905, Los Angeles, CA 90025, USA; [b] Alinsod Institute for Aesthetic Vulvovaginal Surgery, South Coast Urogynecology, Inc. 31852 Coast Highway, Suite 203, Laguna Beach, CA 92651, USA
* Corresponding author.
E-mail address: red@urogyn.org

Clin Plastic Surg 49 (2022) 455–471
https://doi.org/10.1016/j.cps.2022.06.007

only as good as the experienced surgeon. There are many preferred techniques yielding beautiful results, such as a central wedge technique,[6] modified V-wedge technique (V plasty),[7–9] de-epithelization,[10,11] laser labiaplasty,[12] and radiofrequency (RF) labiaplasty. The RF technique will be described in greater detail in this chapter.

Etiology for Hypertrophic Labia Minora and Hood Reduction

It must be clearly stated to the patient and understood that the anatomic variations in width, length, and symmetry are typically within the normal realm of accepted variations. However, when asked why hypertrophic labias occur, the answer is typically multifactorial, such as childbirth, hormonal causes, aging, and often times genetic and congenital.[5,13] Here are examples of the range of normal (Fig. 1).

Can labiaplasty surgery be combined with other gynecologic procedures or cosmetic surgeries?

Labiaplasty is easily paired with other plastic surgery procedures or other gynecologic procedures, such as hysterectomy, bladder slings, and anterior and posterior repairs, vaginoplasties, and perineoplasties.

Basic anatomy

Proper identification of the anatomy is the cornerstone for success in becoming a master genital surgeon. All anatomic variations should be well documented in your notes and in preoperative pictures.

The bilateral mucocutaneous folds between the labia majora and vulvar vestibule are called the nymphae or labia minora.[5,14,15] The labia minora are sensitive to touch during stimulation because of the erectile connective tissue and rich nerve endings (Fig. 2). With sexual arousal, the labia minora will become engorged with blood and appear edematous.[16]

The labia minora split anteriorly to encircle the clitoris forming the clitoral hood and the frenulum of the clitoris. The posterior ends of the labia minora terminate below the clitoris as they become linked together by a skin fold called the frenulum of the labia minora. Where the frenulum and the clitoral hood above it merge is a region called the frenular crease typically found 1 to 2 cm below and lateral to the clitoris. It is not found in textbooks but has been used by Alinsod and others as a landmark to achieve precision and symmetry. Anatomy varies widely and, in some instances, there are dual or almost absent frenulum (Fig. 3).

When operating on the prepuce (clitoral hood), it is important to stay superficial and lateral to the clitoral glans. An understanding of the dorsal nerve of the clitoris is critical to prevent iatrogenic injuries. The pudendal nerve will branch into 3 main branches: the dorsal nerve for the clitoris, the perineal nerve for the external genitalia, and the inferior rectal nerve. The dorsal nerve of the clitoris provides the afferent part for clitoral erection. In addition to the dorsal nerve of the clitoris, the clitoris's cavernous tissue is innervated by the cavernous nerves from the uterovaginal plexus. The two cords of the dorsal nerve of the clitoris terminate 1 cm short of the glans of the clitoris. The shaft of the clitoris is medial to where we typically perform our clitoral hood reduction and is deeper relative to our surgical area. Clitoral hood surgical reduction is akin to a skinning vulvectomy and is very superficial. Risk of clitoral nerve injury is exceptionally low for the knowledgeable labial surgeon.

The blood supply to the labia minora originates from the pudendal artery, including the dorsal artery of the clitoris. Small perforating branches can be found in the labial tissues top to bottom with the ones in the lower third of the labia minora being most problematic for bleeding, bruising, and hematomas (see Fig. 3). Most bleeding sites for labial surgery are easily controlled with electrocautery though occasional suturing may be needed.

The nerve supply to the labia minora and majora originate from the pudendal nerve and become the dorsal labial nerves. This includes the clitoral nerve (Figs. 4 and 5).

Indications

There has been a significant increase in patients seeking surgical correction of the labia minora and clitoral hood reduction. According to the American Society of Aesthetic Plastic Surgeons 2017 statistics, requests for labiaplasty have increased by 217.2% from 2012 to 2017. This significant increase in desire to modify the appearance of the labia minora and clitoral hood may be associated with trends in pubic hair removal as well as increased awareness and discussion through social media and other platforms.

Although variations in appearance are for the most part considered within normal anatomy, the labia minora vary widely in length, thickness, and symmetry.

Basic guidelines for genital esthetics include the following: (1) symmetric labia minora that do not protrude past the labia majora, especially when standing; and (2) a clitoral hood that is reasonably short and nonprotuberant without extra folds.

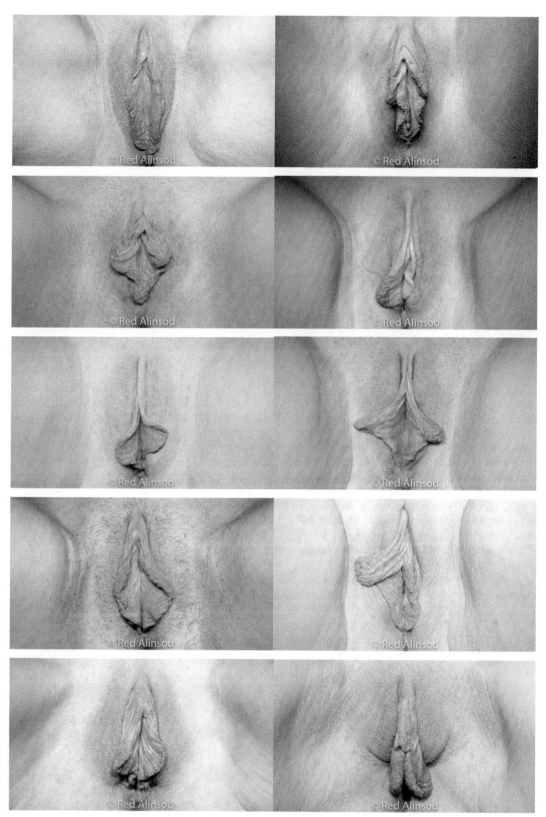

Fig. 1. Normal hypertrophic labia minora and hood examples. (*Courtesy of* Red Alinsod, MD, Laguna Beach, CA.)

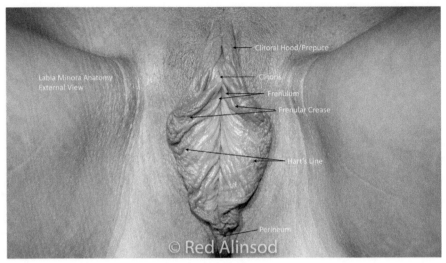

Fig. 2. External vulvar anatomy. (*Courtesy of* Red Alinsod, MD, Laguna Beach, CA.)

Labia minora reduction surgery is performed for reasons of aesthetics or functionality but for most patients it is a combination of both.

There are no absolute contraindications to this procedure. However relative contraindication includes active gynecologic infections and malignancy.[16]

Miklos and Moore: Patients' indications for pursuing surgery. *J Sex Med* 2008; 5:1492 to 1495.[14] In a review by Miklos and Moore, it was revealed 131 patients had undergone a labia reduction surgery: Group I—those who received labia reduction surgery for strictly aesthetic reasons equaled 37% (49/131); Group II—those seeking the surgery strictly for functional impairment equaled 32% (42/131); and Group III—those seeking the surgery for both functional and aesthetic reasons equaled 31% (40/131).

The most common reasons for functional reduction of the labia minora are for recurrent urinary tract infections, hygiene, chronic chafing and irritation during physical activity, labial trauma from childbirth, and a pulling effect leading to insertional dyspareunia. Many women also undergo this type of surgery for aesthetics and confidence issues, such as not liking the bulge under their clothing, asymmetric labias or having to worry about protruding labia in swimsuits or feeling embarrassed during sexual activity.

As indications overlap, most labiaplasties are performed for both a medical therapeutic procedure and cosmetic procedure.

It is important to note that proper screening for body dysmorphic disorder is imperative and refusal to perform surgery and recommendation for proper counseling is vital.

When performing labia minora surgery, a clitoral hood reduction (CHR) is often recommended. The purpose of a CHR is to allow for a debulking and removal of excess and often asymmetrical redundant prepuce on the lateral edges. The most

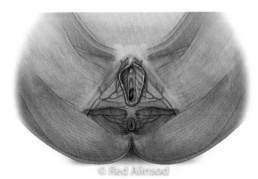

Fig. 3. Vascular supply. (*Courtesy of* Red Alinsod, MD, Laguna Beach, CA.)

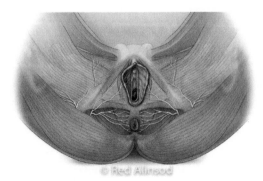

Fig. 4. Nerve supply. (*Courtesy of* Red Alinsod, MD, Laguna Beach, CA.)

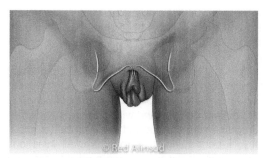

Fig. 5. Clitoral nerve supply. (*Courtesy of* Red Alinsod, MD, Laguna Beach, CA.)

common indication for a CHR is aesthetics as medical-specific indications are less defined.

Goodman[1] defines the goal of this reduction as improving sexual arousal by revealing more of the clitoris. Intuitively this makes sense but no definite studies have been done to confirm this theory. Care must be taken not to unhood the clitoris, which may result in hypersensitivity.

Many authors, including our clinical experience, have reported that a trim curvilinear labiaplasty resection method with a reduction of the labia minora relative to the prominence of the clitoral hood would result in the appearance of being top heavy and would lead to a dissatisfied overall aesthetic outcome for the patient. A micropenis appearance can occur. REFERENCE Therefore, it has been our experience that most labiaplasty minora need to address and consider a clitoral hood reduction at the same time.

Patient evaluation

It is always preferred to have a consultation days before the procedure. This allows for the patient to understand what she is about to undergo and digest the information presented to her before commencing the procedure. However, same-day consultations or virtual consultations followed by a procedure are acceptable as well. The patient evaluation is a great time for both the surgeon and the patient to truly understand what is desired along with setting realistic expected outcomes.

A simple mirror during your physical evaluation is a great tool for mutual decision making and in-depth conversation about the anatomy and realistic expectations. For example, Ms. Jones comes in for uneven and protruding labia minora that cause discomfort during intercourse and feeling insecure about her labia appearance when she is intimate. During the physical examination using a mirror to help the patient view what you are discussing, a decision is made that in addition to helping with symmetry, labia reduction and removal of the darkened edges of the labia are

the other outcomes. A clitoral hood, although not bothersome, should be reduced in size to maintain a symmetric look with the reduction in size of the labias in most instances.

Preoperative Recommendation and Planning

This is the time when a full medical screening for general health, STIs, pregnancy status, anxiety, and establishing a clear understanding of the procedure with realistic expectations and potential complications are thoroughly discussed with the patient. In addition to a verbal discussion of how best to prepare for surgery, we offer our patients a written guideline of preoperative instructions as seen below.

Preoperative preparation for labiaplasty surgery

1. Quitting smoking for a minimum of 4 weeks prior and 3 to 4 weeks after surgery will decrease wound complications by up to 50%.
2. No aspirin or nonsteroidal anti-inflammatory drugs (NSAIDs) should be taken. NSAIDs should be discontinued 7 to 10 days before surgery although Tylenol is acceptable.
3. Discontinue fish oils 7 to 10 days before surgery.
4. We recommend no alcohol 48 hours before the procedure.
5. We recommend starting Arnica or Bromelain 2 days before the procedure and a few days post procedure as a gentle anti-inflammatory.
6. We recommend trimming all pubic hair short around the labias. Avoid shaving or waxing before surgery.
7. Wear loose-fitting comfortable clothes on the day of surgery.
8. Start prophylactic antiviral medications before surgery for history of herpes simplex virus.
9. Must have a driver to take you home from the office or surgery center if any sedation was used.
10. If the procedure is done in an office setting with local anesthesia, we recommend a light meal before surgery and plenty of hydration.

Patient positioning

Patients are placed in a low lithotomy position with proper leg, calf, and ankle support.

We recommend a motorized bed to allow for optimum positioning and visibility for this procedure (**Fig. 6**).

Anesthesia

Almost all labial surgeries are done awake and in the office without an intravenous line. We recommend the patient arrive 1 h before the procedure.

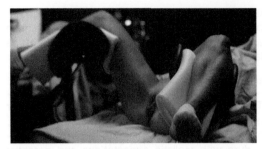

Fig. 6. Leg support. (*Courtesy of* Red Alinsod, MD, Laguna Beach, CA.)

This allows for any paperwork that needs to be completed. It also allows us to review and sign the consents if not done before the day of surgery. We typically recommend all consents be completed in the preoperative consultation. If performed under local anesthesia, we typically will give an anxiolytic such as 1 mg tablet of lorazepam to be administered 30 minutes before starting the procedure in addition to an oral or intramuscular narcotic. Examples are Dilaudid or Demerol. We also recommend applying a numbing cream such as an EMLA cream or compounded numbing cream (30%–35% BLT or bupivacaine/lidocaine/tetracaine) to the area 30 to 60 minutes before the procedure. In some instances, we use Compazine or Zofran as needed. We use a predictive permeation device for about 15 min to drive the numbing cream deeper into the skin. Predictive permeation, also known as dermoelectroporation, opens up the water channels and pushes in the BLT deeper under the skin to improve the numbing effect (**Fig. 7**).

Once proper markings are made, for local procedures, I recommend a mixture of 1% lidocaine with epinephrine 50/50 with 1% marcaine plain buffered with sodium bicarbonate. Another simple option is 0.25% marcaine/bupivacaine with epinephrine buffered with 1 cc sodium bicarbonate to reduce the burning sensation felt upon injection.

Most patients need about 4 to 6 cc of local numbing to achieve the levels needed to proceed without any pain. Keeping the amount of numbing to a minimum is vital and will minimize any disruption of the surgical site and allow for better accuracy in performing the procedure. All injections are recommended to be done medial to the side of surgical dissection on both the medial and lateral aspects of the labia and beneath the clitoral hood as needed (**Figs. 8–11**). The crease between the minora and majora is the ideal location to inject. A 1.5-inch 30-gauge needle works best. I also usually recommend numbing the patient at the end of the case for prolonged comfort. Exparel (liposome-coated bupivacaine) postoperative can give up to 3 days of pain control and is excellent for the traveling patient. Use at the end of the case avoids tissue distortion.

Markings
Marking the patient properly and clearly before starting the local numbing injections that swell and distort the anatomy is crucial. Once the markings are performed, trust and follow them. A proper disposable sterile surgical marking pen should be used with every new case (**Fig. 12**).

When marking the labia minora, we recommend starting laterally and below the frenulum and extending the marking inferiorly till the desired look is achieved. Do not place any pulling tension on the labia as you are marking this will lead to misinterpretation on the amount of resection needed and subsequently over-resection of the labias. Markings should be done on relaxed and untugged labias (**Figs. 13–19**).

It should be noted that significantly large tissue retraction occurs in the upper one-third of the labia minora and therefore a tapering-down incision is recommended. You need to pay close attention

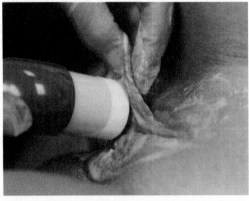

Fig. 7. Predictive permeation. (*Courtesy of* Red Alinsod, MD, Laguna Beach, CA.)

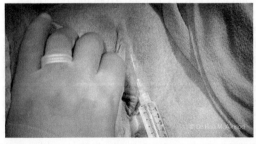

Fig. 8. Start at the crease between the labia minora and majora. (*Courtesy of* Red Alinsod, MD, Laguna Beach, CA.)

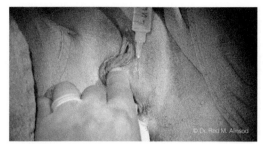

Fig. 9. Inject small drops to avoid distortion of anatomy. (*Courtesy of* Red Alinsod, MD, Laguna Beach, CA.)

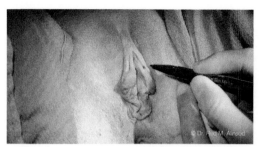

Fig. 13. Start at the frenular crease both medial and lateral. (*Courtesy of* Red Alinsod, MD, Laguna Beach, CA.)

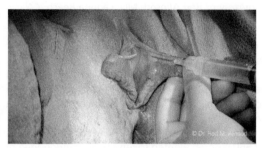

Fig. 10. Inject on the medial aspect at the frenulum, under the hood, and downward. (*Courtesy of* Red Alinsod, MD, Laguna Beach, CA.)

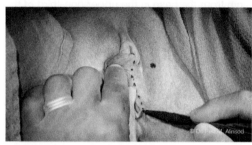

Fig. 14. Lateral dots start below the frenulum. (*Courtesy of* Red Alinsod, MD, Laguna Beach, CA.)

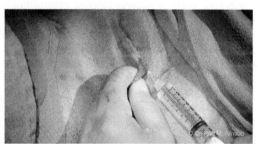

Fig. 11. Inject under the lateral clitoral hood. (*Courtesy of* Red Alinsod, MD, Laguna Beach, CA.)

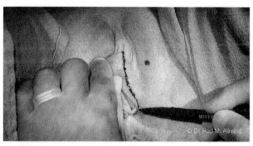

Fig. 15. Connect the dots. (*Courtesy of* Red Alinsod, MD, Laguna Beach, CA.)

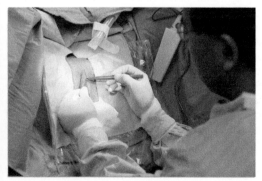

Fig. 12. Use a sterile surgical marker. (*Courtesy of* Red Alinsod, MD, Laguna Beach, CA.)

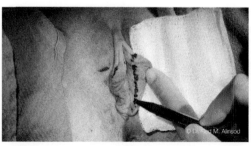

Fig. 16. Medial markings below frenular crease. (*Courtesy of* Red Alinsod, MD, Laguna Beach, CA.)

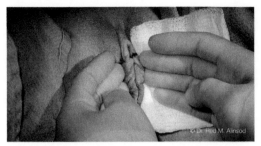

Fig. 17. Kiss the edges for symmetry. (*Courtesy of* Red Alinsod, MD, Laguna Beach, CA.)

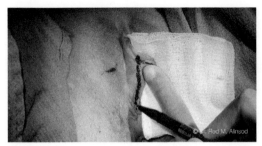

Fig. 19. Right lateral line. Do not pull on the edges while marking. The right-handed surgeon has a tendency to pull on the right labia, which results in aggressive markings that can result in an amputated appearance specially in the top third of the labia. (*Courtesy of* Red Alinsod, MD, Laguna Beach, CA.)

to staying above Hart's line which is approximately 1.5 cm from the base in the upper one-third of the labia. The medial side of the labia is also marked, and we recommend kissing both medial sides to get a proper estimation of symmetry bilaterally. The markings should be made according to the type of labiaplasty a patient desires. The 3 most common variations will be described here.

The Rim Look labiaplasty involves a curve linear excision of only the darkened pigmentation on the rim of the labia. It is the most conservative labial reduction. The Hybrid Look is the most commonly performed type of labiaplasty and is a middle-of-the-road look between the rim appearance and the Barbie labiaplasty (**Figs. 20** and **21**). It leaves a small amount of labia at or below the level of the labia majora.3.

The Barbie Look labiaplasty, coined by Dr. Red Alinsod, removes nearly all of the labia minora and is close to an amputation appearance.3 It looks to create a petite and clam shell appearance that is very comfortable. It works well if there is adequate labia majora puffiness. It is requested by many athletes and fit women who do not want to adjust themselves all day or do not want to outline their labia in tight exercise clothing or swimsuits. We recommend extensive surgical experience performing this type of labiaplasty along with extensive and detailed patient

counseling before performing a Barbie labiaplasty (see **Figs. 53** and **54**).

In a study of 238 women considering labial reduction, 98% sought a labia minora reduction to the level of or below the level of the labia majora.[17]

According to the Miklos and Moore study, 97% of 550 women wanted to remove the dark edges of their labia minora.[17]

The technique we use in marking our clitoral hood and prepuce is based on Dr. Red Alinsod's recommended technique for hood reduction.[3] A 6 to 8 mm vertical midline strip of clitoral hood skin over the central axis of the clitoral hood body is spared. A line is drawn medially preserving 5 to 6 mm as it is attached to the labia minora, we like to call that spared area of clitoral hood the "bridge" and connecting along the lateral edge of the interlabial sulcus.

Surgical technique (LP and clitoral hood reduction)

It is often necessary to reinforce the markings before commencing the surgical dissection. Before discussing the technique, I would like to highlight that meticulous hemostasis is imperative for minimizing bruising and hematoma formation and therefore improving your final outcome. It is also important to remember that when operating on the labia minora a little goes a long way due to the tendency of significant tissue retraction. For this reason when performing your initial surgical markings, my recommendation is to not be fooled by only focusing on the medial mucosal aspect of the labia minora which appears longer than the lateral interlabial fold.

We recommend starting with the more challenging side first and always remembering that if unsure, taking less tissue and staying at or above Hart's line will always pay off as a revision to trim

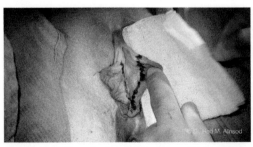

Fig. 18. Post kiss of edges. (*Courtesy of* Red Alinsod, MD, Laguna Beach, CA.)

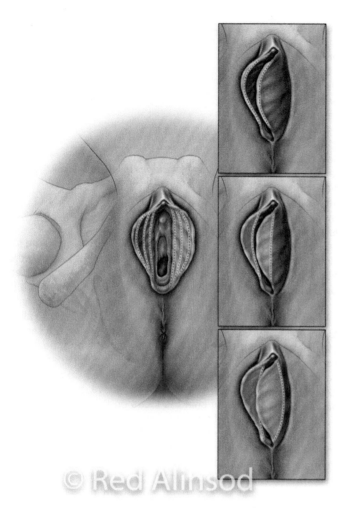

Fig. 20. Illustrated from the top are the Rim, Hybrid, and Barbie Look markings. (*Courtesy of* Red Alinsod, MD, Laguna Beach, CA.)

more tissue is far better than having to deal with an overly resected labium.

Most surgeons performing in office labiaplasties prefer to use an RF pinpoint instrument that allows for precision incisions, minimal lateral spread and some degree of hemostasis. However, many modalities are used with great results such as Metzenbaum scissors, lasers, and scalpel instruments.

Currently in the United States, there are three RF systems currently used for RF pinpoint tip for excision. These are the Ellman Surgitron and Pelleve system and the new Soniquence system released in 2021. Typically, a cutting mode of 10 to 15 W is used for the excision and a blend or coagulation mode of 20 to 25 W.

A great advantage of using the pinpoint needle tip is that the angle of the pinpoint tip can be easily changed to accommodate a change in the degree of direction when cutting into the interstitial tissue of the labia minora.

A recommended technique to minimize the thickness and debulk the labia is to cut at a 45-degree angle into the middle of the labia minora to create a small canal allowing for a debulking effect when reapproximating the edges of the labia.

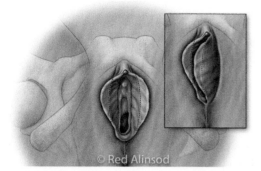

Fig. 21. Markings for an average labial reduction Rim Look. (*Courtesy of* Red Alinsod, MD, Laguna Beach, CA.)

Hence, the term canal incision has been used by Alinsod in his programs.

Once the excision is made along the predetermined marking, hemostasis is imperative. Cautery is ideal in a pinpoint technique (ie, Colorado tip) as opposed to spraying the surface area with the bovie. As an alternative, bipolar RF systems are used once the initial incision has been done to achieve very dry surgical fields (**Figs. 22–29**).

Once meticulous hemostasis is achieved, it should be noted that cauterization leads to increased tissue shrinkage and retraction and therefore one must take this into consideration when making markings and using the cautery device. After completing incision and excision, refinements are performed to ensure edge matching. The smoothing of rough and irregular edges can be performed using the "feathering" technique using the same pinpoint tip popularized by Alinsod.

One of the advantages of having the patient awake is the ability to enlist her approval on the amount of tissue removed. Before starting the incision closure, hand the patient a mirror so she can assess and approve the degree of tissue removed but only if she is feeling comfortable to do so.

We recommend a layered closure to close any dead space (a crucial step in minimizing any hematoma formation).

The initial and deepest layer is closed using a 4 to 0 or 5 to 0 monofilament suture such as Monocryl. We recommend using a noncutting needle, such as a small half circle (SH)-tapered needle. We typically start from the most cephalad portion of the incision below the frenulum and run the suture in an inverted mattress technique (**Figs. 30–32**).

We recommend this type of suture due to the extended delayed breakdown and recommend closing the deepest layer of both labias first. This will allow the surgeon the option for any minor adjustment needed before the final closure of the labia. The second layer closure is typically performed using a synthetic absorbable suture

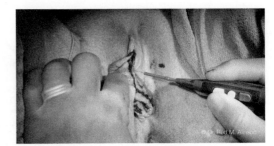

Fig. 23. 45 Degree incisions to create a "canal". (*Courtesy of* Red Alinsod, MD, Laguna Beach, CA.)

composed of polyglycolic acid sutures such as polyglactin 910 (Vicryl).

It is acceptable to use a Vicryl Rapide suture for accelerated suture breakdown but only on the very last layer. Again, a tapered SH needle is preferred over a cutting needle and a 5 to 0 Vicryl suture is recommended. The second layer closure is typically another layer of subcuticular closure to align the edges or a final layer of loosely tied but secure interrupted Vicryl sutures placed along the length of the labia minora. We typically will space them 5 mm apart.

Once the labia minoras have been approximated, we shift the focus on the already marked prepuce if a clitoral hood reduction has been recommended and consented. It has been our experience that the majority of labia minora should undergo at the same time a clitoral hood reduction to maintain the symmetry of the overall look.

Following the premarked markings along the prepuce, we use our RF pinpoint needle with the same settings used for the labiaplasty procedure. Once the excess skin has been removed along the lateral edges of the clitoral hood, close attention is paid to hemostasis using pinpoint cautery and avoiding a spray technique.

The lateral clitoral incisions are closed in a similar multilayer approach. The deepest layer closure consists of a running noninterlocking 5 to 0 Monocryl layer to close any dead space and

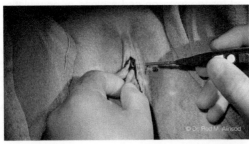

Fig. 22. Pinpoint RF incision. RF, radiofrequency. (*Courtesy of* Red Alinsod, MD, Laguna Beach, CA.)

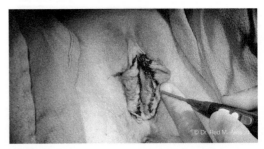

Fig. 24. 45 Degree incision from the medial aspect to create the "canal". (*Courtesy of* Red Alinsod, MD, Laguna Beach, CA.)

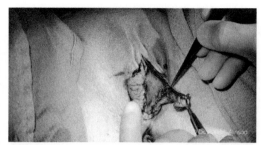

Fig. 25. Bipolar cautery control of bleeding and excision. (*Courtesy of* Red Alinsod, MD, Laguna Beach, CA.)

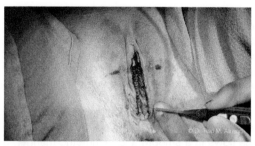

Fig. 29. Using the RF pinpoint tip for refinements and feathering. RF, radiofrequency. (*Courtesy of* Red Alinsod, MD, Laguna Beach, CA.)

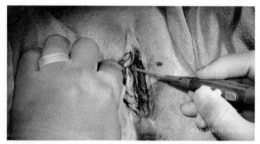

Fig. 26. Pinpoint RF incision into the opposite labia at a 45-degree angle. RF, radiofrequency. (*Courtesy of* Red Alinsod, MD, Laguna Beach, CA.)

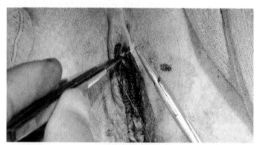

Fig. 30. Deep closure with 5-0 Monocryl suture. (*Courtesy of* Red Alinsod, MD, Laguna Beach, CA.)

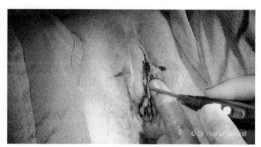

Fig. 27. Pinpoint RF incision from the lateral side at a 45-degree angle for debulking. RF, radiofrequency. (*Courtesy of* Red Alinsod, MD, Laguna Beach, CA.)

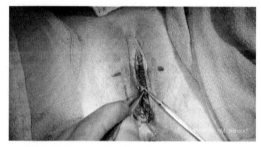

Fig. 31. Inverted mattress suturing. (*Courtesy of* Red Alinsod, MD, Laguna Beach, CA.)

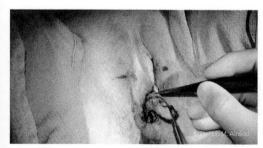

Fig. 28. Bipolar cautery to control bleeding and excise the labia. (*Courtesy of* Red Alinsod, MD, Laguna Beach, CA.)

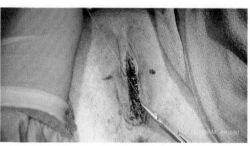

Fig. 32. 5-0 Vicryl interrupted suturing. (*Courtesy of* Red Alinsod, MD, Laguna Beach, CA.)

bring the edges closer together. Once the initial layer is closed, it is a good time to pause and reassess the incision for any small modifications and edits. This is typically followed by a final layer of running a noninterlocking layer using 5 to 0 Vicryl or gently secured interrupted sutures using a 5 to 0 Vicryl (**Figs. 33–48**).

When placing your final layer, it is crucial to properly line the angle downward so that each side flows in a smooth and symmetric manner. 5 to 0 Vicryl or Vicryl Rapide for this layer is perfectly acceptable. It should be noted that both the labiaplasty minora and clitoral hood final layer closure should be gently and loosely tied to minimize tissue strangulation and the anticipation of tissue swelling. Loosely tied sutures will also prevent the scalloped or stair-stepped appearance.

Postoperative instructions

The advantage of combining a clitoral hood reduction with a labiaplasty minora is that the recovery, healing time, and instructions are very similar thereby making it a great combination procedure both for the patient and surgeon.

For both procedures, a detailed discussion and explanation of expectations during the acute recovery stage is vital. I will refer to the first few days of these procedures as the Frankenstein period due to significant bruising and asymmetric swelling that often may occur and frighten the patient. Detailed postoperative instructions are reviewed and given to the patient. We strongly recommend icing every 15 minutes of every hour, when possible, for the first 48 to 72 hours and minimizing excessive walking. We also encourage Arnica, Bromelain, and other anti-inflammatory aids to be taken during this time period. No exercise or heavy lifting is recommended for the first 4 weeks.

Showering is permitted with gentle daily cleansing using soap and water in a cupping-like fashion. We do not recommend taking hot baths

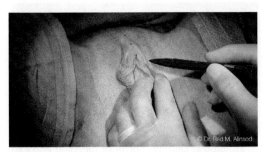

Fig. 34. Marking the midline for a clitoral hood reduction using dots. (*Courtesy of* Red Alinsod, MD, Laguna Beach, CA.)

or soaking in sitz baths for the first 4 weeks as these tend to weaken the suture integrity.

As the sutures start to dissolve many patients report a slightly odorous discharge that may be interpreted as an infection. During this stage of suture lysis, many patients report significant pruritus of the suture line, and an antihistamine is often recommended for this period of the healing. Topical diphenhydramine (Benadryl cream) works very well without sedation. In most cases infections are rare, however, if clinically appropriate culture and treatment for infection is recommended. We encourage the patient to come to the office 2 weeks after surgery for an examination and trimming of sutures if wound edges are healing properly.

Most patients will resume full physical activity including intercourse by week 6, but we recommend if possible, seeing the patient before allowing for intercourse to occur. If there is suturing at the introitus then massage of the suture line is recommended to prevent tearing and pain. Softening of this area with gentle finger massage for 1 to 2 weeks works well.

Although week 6 is often used as a term for complete healing, we recommend making it clear to the patient that the incision itself will soften and be fully healed by the fourth month postprocedure.

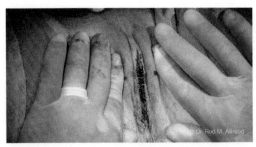

Fig. 33. Final examination of labia minora. (*Courtesy of* Red Alinsod, MD, Laguna Beach, CA.)

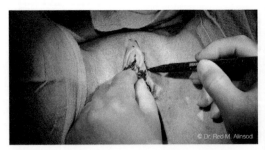

Fig. 35. Marking the lateral border right on the crease. (*Courtesy of* Red Alinsod, MD, Laguna Beach, CA.)

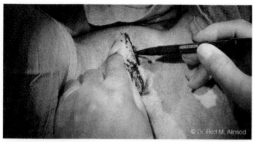

Fig. 36. Marking the top ridge of the clitoral hood. (*Courtesy of* Red Alinsod, MD, Laguna Beach, CA.)

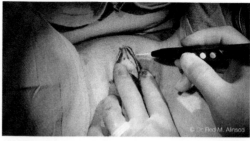

Fig. 40. Incision into the top ridge of the left clitoral hood. (*Courtesy of* Red Alinsod, MD, Laguna Beach, CA.)

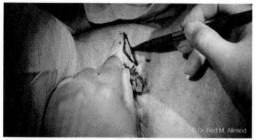

Fig. 37. Completing the elliptical lateral markings on the left. Note the "bridge" separating the edge of the clitoral hood marking and the labial marking. Keep this at least 1 cm wide. (*Courtesy of* Red Alinsod, MD, Laguna Beach, CA.)

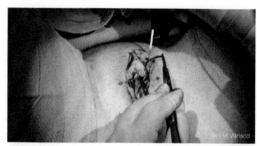

Fig. 41. Skinning excision of the left lateral clitoral hood. (*Courtesy of* Red Alinsod, MD, Laguna Beach, CA.)

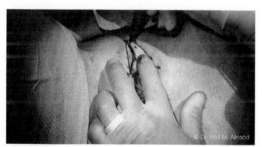

Fig. 38. Marking the top ridge of the opposite side of the clitoral hood. (*Courtesy of* Red Alinsod, MD, Laguna Beach, CA.)

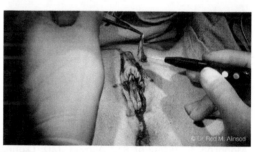

Fig. 42. Left lateral clitoral hood excision completed. (*Courtesy of* Red Alinsod, MD, Laguna Beach, CA.)

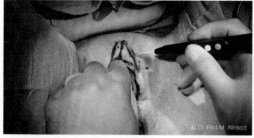

Fig. 39. Gentle and light touch RF incision of the left lateral clitoral hood border. (*Courtesy of* Red Alinsod, MD, Laguna Beach, CA.)

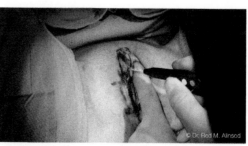

Fig. 43. Right lateral clitoral hood incision. (*Courtesy of* Red Alinsod, MD, Laguna Beach, CA.)

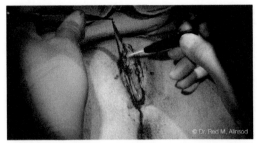

Fig. 44. Right lateral clitoral hood excision complete. (*Courtesy of* Red Alinsod, MD, Laguna Beach, CA.)

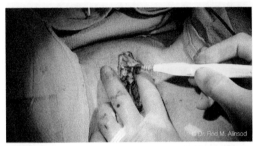

Fig. 45. Hemostasis with standard cautery. (*Courtesy of* Red Alinsod, MD, Laguna Beach, CA.)

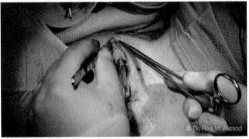

Fig. 46. Inverted mattress sutures with 4-0 or 5-0 Monocryl. (*Courtesy of* Red Alinsod, MD, Laguna Beach, CA.)

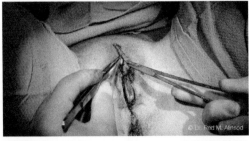

Fig. 47. Skin and fascial edges approximated gently. (*Courtesy of* Red Alinsod, MD, Laguna Beach, CA.)

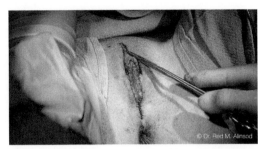

Fig. 48. Interrupted 5-0 Vicryl sutures placed loosely to approximate the edges. (*Courtesy of* Red Alinsod, MD, Laguna Beach, CA.)

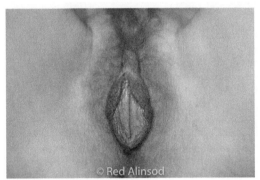

Fig. 49. Rim labiaplasty before. (*Courtesy of* Red Alinsod, MD, Laguna Beach, CA.)

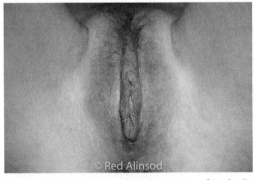

Fig. 50. Rim labiaplasty after. (*Courtesy of* Red Alinsod, MD, Laguna Beach, CA.)

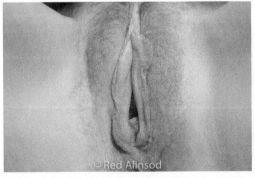

Fig. 51. Hybrid labiaplasty before. (*Courtesy of* Red Alinsod, MD, Laguna Beach, CA.)

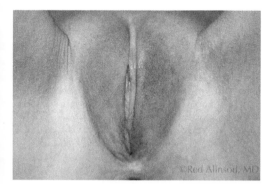

Fig. 52. Hybrid labiaplasty after. (*Courtesy of* Red Alinsod, MD, Laguna Beach, CA.)

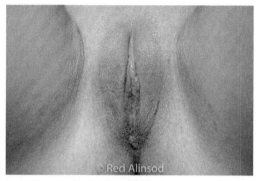

Fig. 54. Barbie look labiaplasty after. (*Courtesy of* Red Alinsod, MD, Laguna Beach, CA.)

Given the nature and sensitivity of these types of procedures, we strongly recommend careful follow-up and being easily accessible to your patients. In our practice, we recommend the initial postoperative follow-up at 1 week and no more than 2 weeks. For patients living far away, we recommend a postoperative virtual consultation.

Postoperative complications
Although complications and adverse events are low, they can range from 2.65%, 12% to 6%.[7]

We highly recommend that the following potential complications be included in your consent for surgery and reviewed with the patient preoperatively.

These complications can include postoperative infection,[13] hematoma,[18] premature suture absorption, wound breakdown, asymmetry, and excessive skin retraction leading to dyspareunia and localized pain. However, the most concerning is overcorrection of the labia minora with a potential for amputation.[3]

Many of these complications are avoided by adhering to the following recommendations:

- Strict adherence to postoperative instructions minimizing excessive walking and lifting
- Using the proper size and material of the suture; Monofilament is a must for the deep layers and avoids premature auto lysis. 5 to 0 Monocryl works well for this layer.
- Avoiding scalloping by placing little tension on the tissue when tying the final layer of the suture line; 5 to 0 Vicryl works well for this top layer.
- Respecting Hart's line and staying surgically conservative if need be
- Keeping the legs together at the knees as much as possible in the first 2 weeks; we affectionately call this "Velcro knees" in our practice
- Avoidance of knee and hip bends for the first month

We recommend listening carefully to patients both preoperatively and postoperatively.

If a revision is recommended, we normally recommend delaying any revision for at least 3 months post-procedure.

Overall, studies have shown high patient satisfaction rates for labiaplasty and clitoral hood reduction procedures with improved aesthetic and functional outcomes. Of 177 patients who had labiaplasty and or clitoral hood reduction, 97.2% were satisfied overall with the outcomes.[7]

Below are examples of Before and After of Rim, Hybrid, and Barbie Look labiaplasties (Figs. 49–54):

SUMMARY

- The most common approach and easiest learning curve to a labiaplasty minora procedure among both gynecologists and plastic surgeons is the curve linear approach.
- The curve linear approach allows for a bigger degree of reduction in length and thickness of

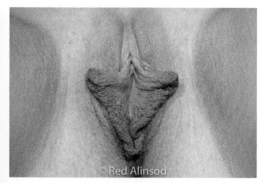

Fig. 53. Barbie look labiaplasty before. (*Courtesy of* Red Alinsod, MD, Laguna Beach, CA.)

the labia minora as opposed to a V-wedge resection. In addition, the curve linear approach allows for removal of the often-present hyperpigmented area and wrinkling on the rim of the labia minora.

- Most labiaplasty minora will need in addition a clitoral hood reduction to maintain symmetry. Therefore, we recommend the patient be given a mirror to observe and discuss the overall look of her vulva.

- When first starting the learning curve for a labiaplasty procedure with the curve linear method, I recommend erring on the conservative side of tissue removal as to minimize the risk of over-resection and unanticipated tissue retraction leading to a potential for amputation.

- I also always recommend allowing the patient to have an active role by showing them the markings and allowing them to ask any questions before starting the case. This allows for greater mutual decision making.

- Maintain exceptional hemostasis and close all dead space before closing your incision thereby optimizing the final result and decreasing the incidence of hematoma and suture separation.

CLINICS CARE POINTS

- The most common approach and easiest learning curve to a labiaplasty minora procedure among both gynecologists and plastic surgeons is the curve linear approach.

- The curve linear approach allows for a bigger degree of reduction in length and thickness of the labia minora as opposed to a V-wedge resection. In addition, the curve linear approach allows for removal of the often present hyperpigmented area and wrinkling on the rim of the labia minora.

- Most labiaplasty minora will need in addition a clitoral hood reduction to maintain symmetry. Therefore, we recommend the patient be given a mirror to observe and discuss the overall look of her vulva.

- When first starting the learning curve for a labiaplasty procedure with the curve linear method, I recommend erring on the conservative side of tissue removal as to minimize the risk of over-resection and unanticipated tissue retraction leading to a potential for amputation.

- I also always recommend allowing the patient to have an active role by showing them the markings and allowing them to ask any questions before starting the case. This allows for greater mutual decision making.

- Maintain exceptional hemostasis and close all dead space before closing your incision thereby optimizing the final result and decreasing the incidence of hematoma and suture separation.

DISCLOSURE

The Authors have nothing to disclose.

REFERENCES

1. Goodman MP. Female cosmetic genital surgery. Obstet Gynecol 2009;113:154–9.
2. Alinsod R. Overview of vaginal rejuvenation, new frontiers in pelvic surgery. Presented at the annual meeting of the national society of cosmetic physicians and the American academy of cosmetic gynecologist, Las Vegas, NV, 2006.
3. Alinsod R. Awake in office Barbie labiaplasty, awake in office labia majora plasty, awake in office vaginoplasty, awake in office labial revision, sutureless band release, awake in office mesh excision, labia majora Pelleve. Presented at the congress on Aesthetic Vaginal Surgery, Tucson, AZ, 2011.
4. Hodgkinson DJ, Hait G. Aesthetic vaginal labioplasty. Plast Reconstr Surg 1984;74:414–24.
5. Tepper OM, Wulkan M, Matarasso A. Labiaplasty: anatomy, etiology, and a new surgical approach. Aesthet Surg J 2011;31:511.
6. Alter GJ. Aesthetic labia minora and clitoral hood reduction using extended central wedge resection. Plast Reconstr Surg 2008;122:1780.
7. Goodman MP, Placik OJ, Benson RH III, et al. A large multicenter outcome study of female genital plastic surgery. J Sex Med 2010;7(4 Pt 1):1565.
8. Felicio Yde A. Labial surgery. Aesthet Surg J 2007; 27:322.
9. Goodman MP. Female Genital cosmetic and plastic surgery: a review. J Sex Med 2011;8:1813.
10. Choi HY, Kim KT. A new method for aesthetic reduction of labia minora (the deepithelialized reduction of labiaplasty). Plast Reconstr Surg 2000;105:419.
11. Cao YJ, Li FY, Li SK, et al. A modified method of labia minora reduction: the de-epithelialized reduction of the central and posterior labia minora. J Plast Reconstr Aesthet Surg 2012;65:1096.
12. Pardo J, Sola V, Ricci P, et al. Laser labiaplasty of labia minora. Int J Gynaecol Surg Obstet 2016; 93:38.
13. Alter GJ. A new technique for aesthetic labia minora reduction. Ann Plast Surg 1998;40:287.

14. Moore RD, Miklos JR. Vaginal reconstruction and rejuvenation surgery: is there data to support improved sexual function. Am J Cosmet 2012; 29:97.

15. Giraldo F, Gonzalez C, de Haro F. Central wedge lumpectomy with a 90-degree Z plasty for aesthetic reduction of the labia minora. Plast Reconstr Surg 2004;113:1820. discussion 1826.

16. Davidson SP, West JE, Baker CL, et al. Medscape. Labiaplasty and labia minora reduction. Available at. http://emedicine.medscape.com/article/1372175-overview.

17. Miklos JR, Moore RD. Postoperative cosmetic expectations for patients considering labiaplasty surgery: our experience with 550 patients. Surg Technol Int 2011;21:170–4.

18. Solanki NS, Tejero-Trujeque R, Stevens-King A, et al. Aesthetic and functional reduction of the labia minora using the Maas and Hage technique. J Plast Reconstr Aesthet Surg 2010;63:1181.

Vaginal Tightening

Lina Triana, MD, Esteban Liscano

KEYWORDS

• Vagina tightening • Vaginoplasty • Perineoplasty • Vaginal rejuvenation • Colporrhaphy

KEY POINTS

- The natural aging process and pregnancies come with certain body changes that influence overall our performance and the vagina is no different.
- Treating a loose vagina, loose vagina walls, will impact sexual gratification on the woman.
- Female sexual gratification is achieved by friction on the anterior vagina wall.
- It is not enough to tight the vaginal entrance to really impact female sexual gratification.
- When tightening the vagina entrance never leaves an inner introitus smaller than the outer introitus.

INTRODUCTION

The natural aging process and pregnancies come with certain body changes that influence our overall performance and the vagina is no different. With time, earth's gravity force pulls everything down including our internal and external sexual organs making them less firm and loose. This, plus the natural process through which a woman goes through during their pregnancy, impacts her vagina.

When a woman gets pregnant the baby's weight is sustained by the pelvic floor muscles. These same muscles hold the vagina in place. After nine months of the baby's weight being supported by the pelvic floor muscles, once the baby is born and these muscles do not have to hold this extra weight, they end up being loose and cannot keep the vagina's original place and shape (**Fig. 1**).

With these vagina changes that leave the woman with loose vagina walls comes the concept of vagina tightening.

With looser vaginal walls, the woman during sexual intercourse cannot tight her vaginal as before preventing during sexual intercourse that the penis is pushed to the anterior vagina wall where a higher number of sensitivity receptors is present. Less friction on the anterior vagina walls means less sexual gratification for her. Also, loosening of pelvic floor muscles and the vagina walls will influence the bladder position, promoting stress incontinence.

Treating a loose vagina, loose vagina walls, will impact sexual gratification on the woman.[1] Understanding this simple concept is crucial for making a correct surgical plan to our patient.

Only tightening the vagina entrance is no enough to really impact female sexual gratification. When only the entrance is repaired males will benefit from it since for them friction on the penis surface give them sexual gratification, but for women it is more important to improve vagina wall tone overall so that this woman can push harder the penis to her anterior vagina wall during sexual intercourse and achieve sexual gratification.[2]

DEFINITIONS
Vaginoplasty

Vaginoplasty is also called colporrhaphy or vaginal rejuvenation. It is the tightening of the inner vagina walls and can be done on the anterior, posterior, or lateral aspects of the vagina wall.

Perineoplasty

It is the tightening of the vagina entrance.

Vagina Introitus

It is the vagina entrance and is constituted by the outer and inner introitus. The inner introitus is found at the level of the caruncle remnants.

The author has nothing to disclose.
Corpus and Rostrum Surgery Center, Calle 3 Oeste #34-19, Cali, Valle, Colombia, South America
E-mail address: Linatriana@drlinatriana.com

Clin Plastic Surg 49 (2022) 473–478
https://doi.org/10.1016/j.cps.2022.06.008
0094-1298/22/© 2022 Elsevier Inc. All rights reserved.

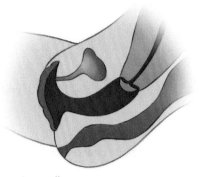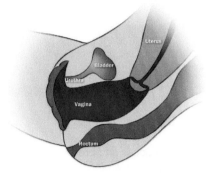

Fig. 1. Loosen vagina walls.

Anatomy

The vagina is a fibromuscular tube which extends from the vestibule to the cervix. The walls of the vagina are in apposition except at the apex where it is held open by the cervix. The vagina takes a slightly S-shaped course, curving at the perineum and cervix.

Vaginal length is approximately 8.4 cm with the angle between the upper and lower vaginal segments averaging 129°. The anterior vaginal length is approximately 6 to 9 cm in comparison with the posterior vaginal length of 8 to 12 cm.

The normal vaginal wall is 2 to 3 mm thick, consisting on four distinct histologic layers: the mucosa which is a nonkeratinized stratified squamous epithelium. Beneath the mucosa is a thin layer of loose connective tissue, the lamina propria. The muscular layer beneath the lamina propria, the vaginalis muscularis consists of smooth muscle, and the layer developed by separating the vaginal epithelium from the muscularis is known as the pubocervical fascia anteriorly and the rectovaginal fascia posteriorly. Adherent to the muscularis is the adventicia; this is an extension of the endopelvic fascia.[3]

ANATOMIC RELATIONSHIPS

Anteriorly, the vagina lies adjacent to and supports the bladder base, and the endopelvic fascia lies between the vagina and bladder (**Fig. 2**).[4]

The urethra is fused with the anterior vagina wall with no intervening adventitial layer. The ureters cross the lateral vaginal fornices.

The posterior vagina is defined by the cul-de-sac of Douglas superiorly, the rectum posteriorly and the perineal body inferiorly.

The rectovaginal septum is an additional layer embryologically derived from fused layers of cul-de-sac peritoneum, which is attached to the posterior surface of the vaginal muscularis.

The vaginal axis is maintained by a combination of muscular and ligamentous support along the length of the vaginal wall.

The pelvis is a basin formed by muscles. The entry is open and round. The back wall is formed by sacrum centrally and the piriformis muscles laterally, the sidewalls are the right and left obturator internus muscles, and the front wall is formed by the back of the pubic bodies and pubis symphysis. The floor is formed by the levator ani muscle complexes and the coccygeus muscles covering the sacrospinous ligaments.[4]

DIAGNOSIS

First, it is important to listen to the patient:
- I would like to feel the same (sexual gratification) than before.
- I feel I cannot tighten my vagina as I did it before.
- During sexual intercourse, it sounds as if air gets into my vagina.
- She refers urinary stress incontinence symptoms.

Second, examine the patient:
- In lithotomy position ask the patient to push, watch for vagina prolapses.
- Observe vaginal mucosa, is it pale or with inflammatory changes.
- Perform an internal vagina examination without lubrication look for looseness at the entrance, the anterior and the posterior vagina walls.

The ideal patient for a vagina tightening procedure is the patient who tells us she does not feel the same during sexual intercourse, feels her vagina is loose and during examination you feel the loss in tone in her internal vagina (a vaginoplasty is needed) and/or her vagina entrance (a perineoplasty is needed) and no big prolapse is found. May woman suffer for urinary stress incontinence,

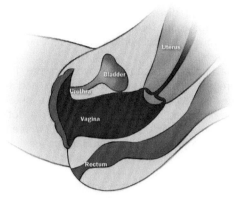

Fig. 2. Vagina relationships.

in them you may find a small prolapse which will be improved by tightening her vagina walls.

CHOOSING THE RIGHT CLINICAL/SURGICAL MANAGEMENT

Patients with not a big vaginal wall looseness or those with urinary stress incontinence that do not want to overcome a surgery and are willing to have several repetitive treatments can be good candidates for a nonsurgical laser vaginal rejuvenation approach.[5] Kegel exercises alone can help but in the author experience will not resolve the problem.

Important to explain what to expect with the different treatment options.[6] When a correct surgical plan is chosen, we will have a happy patient. This is why it is crucial to touch the inner vagina walls during consultation and plan where the tightening procedure will take place. Generally, if the patient mentions she wants to increase sexual gratification a posterior wall tightening is needed and if she refers urinary stress incontinence or if a small prolapse is seen she is a good patient for an upper wall tightening.

If the patient has more than stress incontinence the condition may not be resolved after a vagina tightening procedure.[4,7]

SURGICAL TECHNIQUE
Presurgery

All patients before entering the operating room must have a urine culture and a vaginal smear and also a vaginal cervix cytology to discard urine or vaginal infections and vaginal cervix pathologies.

Complete presurgical blood tests are also done on the patient.

Surgical Technique
Surgery sequence
During the consultation, the ideal surgical plan will be created. If the patient needs tightening on the anterior and posterior vagina walls and on the vagina entrance the preferred surgical sequence will be to start with the anterior tightening, followed by the skin dissection of the perineoplasty, continued by the posterior tightening and finalizing with the suturing of the perineoplasty.

General aspects
The procedure is done under general anesthesia.

Using a labia minora retractor opens the vagina and help with the visualization of the inner aspect of the vagina. This retractor is used for the anterior and posterior vaginal tightening procedures and is not used for the perineoplasty.

The use of a pudendal block improves postsurgical anesthesia. This pudendal block is done on the patient once anesthetized.

The patient will have a urethra catheter that will be introduce once the patient is put to sleep and will be removed before the patient wakes up. In some cases, if the patient cannot have normal urination (urinates with force or experiences urine retention) the urethral catheter will be put back again for several days.

Pudendal block
A pudendal block kit is needed. Identify the ischial spine through a vaginal examination, introduce the needle with its needle holder (come with the pudendal block kit), and lean it over the ischial spine. Aspirate and introduce 5 cm^3 of bupivacaine on each ischial spine. On very thin patients be aware after this block, they can experience difficulties walking due to decreased power on their leg muscles for several hours, this condition will pass away, the patient will just need observation.

Tumescent solution
Tumescent solution is used to decrease bleeding and help hydro-dissection. Tumescent solution is prepared by using 1 cm^3 of epinephrine for each on 1000 cm^3 of saline solution.

Anterior vagina tightening
The uterus is grabbed downwards.

Enough tumescent solution is applied until it ends up with the whitening of the mucosa.

A little bit above where the uterus neck joins with the uterus body a horizontal incision of about 1 cm long is done. The author uses a laser as a cutting device but it can be done without it too.

Three Allis forceps are used, the first one placed 1 cm above the horizontal incision and the other two on the borders of the incision. The use of these three forceps helps us producing tension and helping the surgery for a tent-like mucosal dissection.

Scissors are introduced through the horizontal incision and dissection is done on an upward manner for about 1 cm.

The mucosa is cut vertical on the midline of the elevated flap.

The first Allis forceps is moved upward 1 cm where the mucosa dissection finishes and two more Allis forceps are used, one on each side of the dissected mucosa. The mucosal dissection is continued on an upward manner until the corrugate anterior wall mucosa is reached. To verify the dissection has reached its limit, the surgeon can pull the urethral catheter and feel the dissection is not above the balloon. If the dissection is kept too high and stiches are placed above the balloon (above the detrusor sphincter) the patient can end up with permanent urinary retention.

Blunt dissection is achieved with a gauze along the lateral aspects of the dissected mucosa until no more laxity is found.

Hemostasis is done.

Plication of the fascia is done with a 2-0 vicryl suture in a continuous crossed manner starting on from the inside to the outside (from the uterus neck to the urethral orifice). Remember we have the urethra in the midline of the plication and to keep it out of the way when suturing the needle must be introduce sideways avoiding the midline.

If the patient has urinary stress incontinence, then one or two more stiches will be done above the detrusor sphincter to correct it.

Excess mucosa is resected.

Hemostasis is done.

Anterior wall mucosa is closed by using a 2-0 vicryl suture in a continuous crossed manner starting on from the inside to the outside (from the uterus neck to the urethral orifice).

Posterior vagina tightening

If the patient will have a perineoplasty too, markings of the skin to be resected on the perineal area are done.

The uterus is grabbed upwards.

Enough tumescent solution is applied until it ends up with the whitening of the mucosa.

The previous marked perineal skin is resected.

Three Allis forceps are used, the first one placed 1 cm above the horizontal incision and the other two on the borders of the incision. The use of these three forceps helps us producing tension and helping the surgery for a tent-like mucosal dissection.

Scissors are introduced through the horizontal incision and dissection is done on an upward manner for about 1 cm.

The mucosa is cut vertical on the midline of the elevated flap.

The first Allis forceps is moved upward 1 cm where the mucosa dissection finishes and two more Allis forceps are added, one on each side of the dissected mucosa. The mucosal dissection is continued on an upward manner until where the uterus neck joins with the uterus body. The author uses a laser as a cutting device but it can be done without it too.

Blunt dissection is achieved with a gauze along the lateral aspects of the dissected mucosa until no more laxity is found.

Hemostasis is done.

Plication of the fascia is done with a 2-0 vicryl suture in a continuous crossed manner starting on from the inside to the outside (from the uterus neck to the external introitus). Remember we have the rectum just mm away.

Excess mucosa is resected.

Hemostasis is done.

Posterior wall mucosa is closed by using a 2-0 vicryl suture in a continuous crossed manner starting on from the inside to the outside (from the uterus neck to the external introitus) until the plication finishes.

Perineoplasty

Two mosquito forceps are used to measure the new external introitus and mark the perineal skin to be resected. Very important to make sure that the inner introitus is never smaller than the external one. If we end up with an external introitus small than the inner introitus when the patient has sexual intercourse tearing's can occur in the vagina entrance (**Fig. 3**).

The excess previously marked perineal skin is removed and mucosal dissection starts from the outside to the inside until the previously marked border on the posterior vagina wall.

Blunt dissection is done, on the lateral aspects of the posterior wall and also the pubococcygeal muscle.

Hemostasia y Done

Plication of the fascia is done with a 2-0 vicryl suture in a continuous crossed manner starting on from the inside to the outside (from the uterus neck to the vagina entrance). Generally, this plication stops at the inner introitus level where the pubococcygeal muscles are seen. The plication of these two muscles to the midline is done with at least three sutures (one on the anterior, one on the posterior aspects of the muscle, and one in the midline).

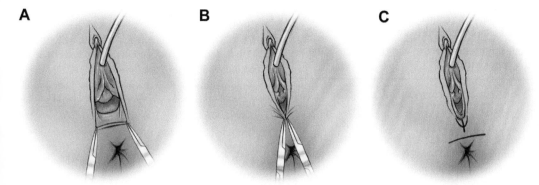

Fig. 3. Marking the new external introitus. (*A*) Marking the excess skin. (*B*) Making sure the external introitus is not smaller than the internal introitus. (*C*) Final markings.

Excess mucosa is resected.

Check hemostasia before start suturing.

The posterior vagina wall mucosa is closed by using a 2-0 vicryl suture in a continuous crossed manner starting on from the inside to the outside (from the uterus neck to the internal introitus).[8]

Suturing is stopped at the internal introitus where remnants of the caruncle, if present, are approximated.

Continuation of the closing is performed with individual sutures all the way from the internal introitus to the external introitus where labia minora joins in the midline and continues to the perineal skin, all with individual vicryl 2-0 sutures.

Postsurgery

If the patient presents urination difficulties after the procedure a ureteral catheter will be put back in place for several days.

For eight days, no friction in the area is advise including not wearing tight cloths.

Cleaning with an antiseptic solution for 3 days is encouraged.

No exercising of sexual intercourse for 6 weeks.

Stiches will fall out with time but if after 3 weeks you can still see them on the external skin they will be removed.

Complications

We must never forget when performing a vagina tightening procedure, we are working only millimeters apart from important structures such as the urethra, the bladder, and the rectus. This is why a fistula connecting these organs can happen.

Bleeding can always be a problem in the area because the vagina is a highly vascularized organ. This is why it is very important to have sufficient tumescent solution not only for helping during dissection but for prevention excessive cauterization and possible perforations.

Tightening the anterior vaginal wall can be more challenging as it represents a higher risk of

damaging the urethra, to prevent the needle must always stay away from the midline when performing the fascia plication.

Postsurgical bleeding can happen, for this packaging with a vagina gauze for several days may be needed.

Some patients can be sensible to opioids derivatives such as fentanyl used during anesthesia or postsurgical medications. If patient experiences urine retention after the procedure send them home with a urethral catheter and the condition is mainly caused by contraction of the detrusor sphincter, sphincter between the bladder and the urethra, send patient home with medication to relax it, such as tamsulosin.

Controversies

Controversies regarding vagina tightening procedures arise from the dilemma: do we need to intervene even when we do not have an evident prolapse.[1] Although today there is not enough scientific evidence to overcome the dilemma, it is clear that patients who seek for these procedures have in common the wiliness to improve sexual gratification, to feel as they used to feel before, so why do not help them with the technology we have today. What is a normal breast, why do plastic surgeons today intervene a not deformed breast and enhance it? Because plastic surgery is all about improving quality of life and this is what we do when we perform to our patient a vagina tightening procedure.

CLINICS CARE POINTS

- Maintain the area as dry as possible for eight days after the procedure.
- No tight clothing for eight days.

- No sexual intercourse or excersicing for six weeks after the procedure.
- Never tighten more the vagina entrance than the inner introitus.

REFERENCES

1. Moore R, Miklos J. Vaginal Reconstruction and Rejuvenation Surgery: Is There Data To Support Improved Sexual Function? The American Journal of Cosmetic Surgery. June 2012. The American Journal of Cosmetic Surgery 29(2):97–113. DOI:10.5992/AJCS-D-12-00002.
2. Nahai F, Kenkel J, Stevens G, et al. The art of aesthetic surgery: principles and techniques, Thieme New York, 3rd edition, Chaper 106 vaginal rejuvenation and perineoplasty: surgical alteration and minimally invasive procedures: part 2 — vaginal tightening: surgical and nonsurgical options. P. 1574–1080.
3. Moore C, Daneshgari F. Vaginal anatomy for the pelvic surgeon. Vaginal surgery for incontinence and prolapse. Springer, New York;2016:3–10.
4. Rogers R. Pelvic floor anatomy: made clear and simple. Urogynecology in primary care: Springer, New York; 2007:11–20.
5. Gaviria J, Lanz J. Laser Vaginal tightening (LVT) evaluation of a novel noninvasive laser treatment for vaginal relaxation syndrome. J Laser Health Acad 2012;1:59–66.
6. Leah M, Racher P, Seth H, et al. Radiofrequency treatment of vaginal laxity after vaginal delivery: nonsurgical vaginal tightening. J Sex Med 2010;7:3088–95.
7. Sohail A. Vaginal anatomy and phisiology. J Pelvic Med Surg 2005;9:263–72.
8. Triana L. Aesthetic vaginal plastic surgery - a practical guide: Springer, New York; 2020.

Mons Pubis Lift (Monsplasty)

Maryam Saheb-Al-Zamani, MA, MD, FRCSC[a,b,*]

KEYWORDS

- Mons pubis lift • Monsplasty • Monspexy • Mons suspension • Liposuction

KEY POINTS

- The mons pubis is a fatty hair-bearing domed unit that is continuous with the lower abdomen and contributes to truncal aesthetics.
- Excess fullness and/or ptosis of the mons pubis from weight fluctuation or aging can result in poor aesthetics, psychosocial and sexual distress, and hygiene issues.
- Assessment of mons pubis aesthetics should involve the evaluation of 3 parameters: (1) fatty fullness, (2) vertical ptosis, and (3) horizontal expansion.
- Based on patient presentation, appropriate surgical correction of the mons may include dermolipectomy, debulking, suspension, and/or horizontal excess correction.
- To avoid overresection and somatosensory issues, monsplasty should position the anterior commissure at the lower edge of the pubic symphysis and tissue should not be resected caudal to the pubic symphysis.

INTRODUCTION

As the anterior-most component of the vulva and continuous with the lower abdomen, the mons pubis can significantly affect truncal aesthetics. Excess adiposity or ptosis of this structure, due to weight fluctuations or aging, can result in notable deformity that can be apparent even clothing, decrease self-esteem, present as a barrier to intimacy, and negatively affect hygiene and sexual function. This article aims to familiarize the reader with relevant anatomy, common aesthetic concerns, as well as a well-rounded overview of described approaches to mons pubis lift (monsplasty). Complications and clinical pearls are discussed to help surgeons avoid potential pitfalls.

Mons Pubis Anatomy

The mons pubis is a triangular unit defined centrally by a hair-bearing slightly domed fatty elevation. It is bound laterally by the inguinal folds, superiorly by the upper extent of pubic hairline and pubohypogastric fold, and continues inferiorly to the labia majora.[1,2] The pubis is the ventral projection of hip bones that fuse centrally via the cartilaginous pubic symphysis. The fatty triangular mass of mons pubis overlies the pubic bone. Similar to the abdomen, the fat layer in the mons can be differentiated into superficial and deep compartments, separated by a superficial fascial layer, which is a continuation of Scarpa's fascia from the abdomen and Colle's fascia in the perineum.[3] Above the superficial fascial layer, the lamellar adipose layer is composed of tightly packed small fat lobules among orthogonal septa. Below the superficial fascial layer, large fat lobules loosely organized in larger septal compartments constitute the areolar adipose layer.[4]

Sensation to the lower abdomen and superior inguinal regions is provided by the anterior cutaneous branch of the iliohypogastric nerve (L1), which arises from the main trunk because it travels between the transversus abdominis and internal

Financial Disclosures/Conflicts of Interest: None.
[a] Private Practice, Toronto, Ontario, Canada; [b] ICLS Plastic Surgery, 1344 Cornwall Road, Oakville, Ontario L6J 7W5, Canada
* ICLS Plastic Surgery, 1344 Cornwall Road, Oakville, Ontario L6J 7W5, Canada.
E-mail address: Maryam.s.zamani@gmail.com

Clin Plastic Surg 49 (2022) 479–487
https://doi.org/10.1016/j.cps.2022.06.003
0094-1298/22/© 2022 Elsevier Inc. All rights reserved.

oblique. Mons pubis (and labia majora) is innervated by the ilioinguinal (L1) and genitofemoral (L1-2) nerves. The ilioinguinal nerve pierces the internal oblique muscle and courses through the inguinal canal and superficial ring to provide sensation to the lower inguinal region, mons pubis, anterior labia majora, and adjacent medial thighs. The genital branch of the genitofemoral nerve arises from the genitofemoral nerve above the inguinal ligament and travels with the round ligament to innervate to the mons pubis and labia majora.[5]

Blood supply to the pubic symphysis and mons region is from branches of the inferior epigastric artery superiorly, the deep external pudendal artery anteriorly, and inferiorly by the dorsal artery of the clitoris, which arises from the internal pudendal artery. The inferior epigastric artery stems from the internal iliac artery, whereas the deep external pudendal artery and internal pudendal artery are tributaries of the femoral artery.[6] Venous drainage is provided by the concomitant veins. Superficial inguinal lymph nodes drain the lower trunk and mons. The dominant cutaneous lymphatic network is located subdermally but eventually pierce Scarpa's fascia to drain into the inguinal nodes within 2 to 3 cm of the inguinal ligament. Additional lymphatic drainage is provided by a deep system overlying fascia that drains the muscles, fascia, and nerves and follows the arterial supply pattern.[7]

Aesthetic Goals and Treatment Indications

In young women, the vertex angle of the mons pubis between the inguinal folds is closer to 60° with minimal fullness. In adulthood, this angle is closer to 90° and the mons has a longer vertical axis and domal fullness. The vulvar commissure is positioned at the lower edge of the pubic symphysis projection. With age and significant weight gain, the mons elongates and presents with a longer horizontal axis and is more obtuse, reaching 100° or more. These changes relate to fatty tissue accumulation, stretch and laxity of the superficial fascia, and expansion of the skin envelope in the vertical plane and, to various degrees, the horizontal plane.[1,8–11] Even after massive weight loss, dysmorphism of the mons pubis commonly remains, leading to aesthetic dissatisfaction, discomfort and poor fit in clothing, and psychosocial distress, and decreased quality of life. Functionally, the hanging mons can result in poor hygiene, local infections, urinary dysfunction, and compromised sexual performance.[9,11]

Treatment goals of mons pubis lift aim to restore the mons to a more youthful contour, commonly necessitating reduction of fatty excess as well as skin removal and suspension superiorly to elevate the mons to its original position and correct overhang over the external genitalia. Careful assessment of mons pubis is key to selecting the correct combination of techniques to achieve sustainable desired results.

Monsplasty can be performed concurrently with other body contouring procedures, including standard abdominoplasty,[8,9,12–15] Fleur-de-Lis abdominoplasty,[16] lower body lift,[4] and thigh lift.[1,17] Failure to recognize and address a full and/or ptotic mons during body contouring procedures can present as exaggeration of the mons deformity against a now flattened abdomen and lead to patient dissatisfaction. Monsplasty may be indicated in isolation if this area has been neglected during previous abdominal contouring.[15]

Assessment

A thorough history and physical examination is pertinent to successful surgical outcome. Specific to the mons pubis lift, patients are asked regarding their aesthetic concerns, hygiene, irritation and infections, sexual and urinary function. The patient is then evaluated in standing position. If the patient has a hanging pannus that will be addressed with concurrent abdominoplasty, pannus elevation is simulated to assess mons fullness, position, and skin excess in isolation. Standard body contouring photograph series as well as views with the pannus lifted are obtained for documentation.

Three grading systems have been described in the literature to discuss mons pubis deformity and treatment planning. The first was The Pittsburg Rating Scale, which assesses fullness versus ptosis to recommend liposuction versus monsplasty.[18] Later classifications by El Khatib[8] in 2010 and Pechevy[19] in 2016 expanded on different stages of mons deformity and provided more detail on surgical treatment recommendations. El Khatib and Pechey both recommend liposuction for treatment of mild mons fullness and arching without associated ptosis. In cases of moderate mons fatty fullness and some degree of ptosis manifesting as partial coverage of the external genitalia, both classification systems recommend liposuction and superior mons skin excision, referred to herein as dermolipectomy, "panniculectomy" by El Khatib and "upper base trapezoid excision" after staged skin removal following abdominoplasty by Pechevy. The third type of mons presentation involved significant fatty accumulation, ptosis, and complete coverage over the external genitalia. El Khatib performs liposuction for debulking, whereas Pechevy recommends direct fat excision as needed to complement liposuction. In addition to debulking and dermolipectomy for vertical excess skin reduction, both authors recognize the need to elevate and anchor the mons to its proper position with permanent suspension sutures. El Khatib places suspension sutures that capture dermis and subcutaneous tissues of the mons flap and anchors them to rectus sheath (dermal-fascial suspension sutures), whereas Pechevy places "pexy" fascial sutures. The fourth type of mons deformity presents as deflation and ptosis, with no excess arching and partial or complete coverage of external genitalia. El Khatib and Pecheby both recommend dermolipectomy and mons suspension. For type 3 and 4 mons deformities, El Khatib also acknowledges that there can be horizontal skin laxity and excess that can require treatment via a central wedge excision. These 3 classification systems are shown in **Table 1**, amended with common terminology to allow comparison.

Approach

Once the parameter(s) contributing to mons deformity have been identified, surgical techniques can be selected and combined to offer best correction for the patient. A simple decision algorithm is demonstrated in **Fig. 1**. Regardless of the classification system used, 3 parameters must be assessed for to adequately treat mons pubis deformity:

- Is there excess mons fullness?
- Is the mons ptotic?
- Is there horizontal expansion in addition to vertical excess and laxity?

Mons skin excision (dermolipectomy) markings. The patient is marked in standing position. Areas of excess fullness of the mons are marked for liposuction and/or direct fat excision. If the mons is ptotic, the nondominant hand is used to elevate the mons, ensuring that the anterior commissure is restored to its normal position at the lower edge of the pubic symphysis and avoiding excessive pull and distortion of the clitoris.[15] Bony landmarks are thereby exposed and can be marked for reference. Additionally, the amount of skin excess requiring excision can be measured and marked. Skin excision, if any, is planned above the hairbearing pubic region, 5 to 8 cm above the commissure.[4,8,9,12,13] The marking is then extended laterally as is typical for the associated abdominoplasty or lower body lift.[4,8] Marques[9] described a more conservative approach to excision of superior mons dermolipectomy, whereby

skin excision of abdominal pannus is planned for and performed separately from mons skin excision. The mons dermolipectomy is planned as a separate trapezoid, where the larger base corresponds to the abdominoplasty horizontal incision, the parallel shorter base is 5 to 7 cm above the commissure, and the oblique sides are marked 1.5 to 2.5 cm above the inguinal folds. Dermolipectomy of the mons is performed after resection of abdominoplasty pannus is completed.[9] This technique can help safeguard against excess skin excision and upward pull of the external genitalia and may be recommended for surgeons new to this procedure. In cases where monsplasty is performed in isolation where either body contouring is not indicated or more likely, the mons was overlooked at the time of the original surgery, a horizontal crescentic excision pattern is placed just below the panniculus fold or in a preexisting abdominoplasty scar.[15]

Mons debulking. Thickness of the tissues of the anterior abdominal wall and mons are compared. If excess fullness of the mons is present, then debulking of the fatty layer is performed for smooth transition by liposuction[8,11,15,19] and/or direct fat excision.[4,9,11–15,19,20] Although there is consensus regarding mons debulking to achieve appropriate contour and transition from the lower abdomen to the pubis, there is controversy regarding the depth from which fat should be removed. Some authors recommend removal of the lamellar fat located above the superficial fascia,[9] whereas others recommend removal of the areolar deep fat located below the superficial fascia and above the muscular abdominal wall.[4,8,14,20] Some address both layers, using liposuction to thin superficial fat layer and enhance skin contraction, and remove fat directly from the deep layer if necessary.[15,19,21]

Surgeons that advocate superficial fat excision do so in order to preserve deep lymphatics and minimize seroma formation.[9] Anatomical studies of the lower trunk lymphatics have demonstrated the presence of 2 systems: a dominant superficial network that drains the skin and subcutaneous fat and a deeper network that drains the fascia, muscles, and nerve. The cutaneous lymphatic system runs subdermally, superficial to Scarpa's fascia for the most part, and piercing Scarpa's fascia to run in the sub-Scarpal plane only within 2 to 3 cm of the inguinal ligament to drain into the superficial inguinal nodes.[7] The deeper lymphatic network is located close to fascial planes and does not exist within adipose tissues.[7,22] As in abdominoplasty, preservation of a thin layer of tissue over the deep fascia (rectus sheath in the abdomen; the Gallaudet fascia in the pubic region)

Table 1
Comparison of 3 described classification systems and suggested treatment algorithms for mons pubis deformity

Pittsburgh Rating Scale (2005)		El Khatib's Classification (2010)		Pechevy's Classification (2016)	
Classification	*Treatment*	*Classification*	*Treatment*	*Classification*	*Treatment*
1: Excess fat	Liposuction	1: Mild excess fat without or with minimal ptosis (no/partial external genitalia coverage)	Liposuction	1: Mild excess fat without or with minimal ptosis (no/partial external genitalia coverage)	Liposuction
2: Ptosis	Monsplasty	2: Moderate excess fat with moderate ptosis (partial external genitalia coverage)	Liposuction + Dermolipectomy ("panniculectomy")	2: Moderate excess fat with moderate ptosis (partial external genitalia coverage)	Liposuction + Dermolipectomy ("upper base trapezoid excision")
3: Significant ptosis (overhang below symphysis)	Monsplasty	3: Significant excess fat with significant ptosis (complete external genitalia coverage)	Liposuction + Dermolipectomy ("panniculectomy") + Mons suspension (dermal-fascial) +/– Horizontal excess reduction (vertical wedge excision)	3: Significant excess fat with significant ptosis (complete external genitalia coverage)	Liposuction + Dermolipectomy ("upper base trapezoid excision") + Direct fat excision ("panniculectomy") + Mons suspension (fascial-fascial; "pexy")
		4: No excess fat with ptosis (partial or complete external genitalia coverage)	+ Dermolipectomy ("panniculectomy") + Mons suspension (dermal-fascial) + Horizontal excess reduction (vertical wedge excision)	4: No excess fat with ptosis (partial or complete external genitalia coverage)	Dermolipectomy ("upper base rapezoid excision") + Mons suspension (fascial-fascial; "pexy")

The descriptions have been adjusted to allow for comparison across the different classification systems. The authors' original terminology is included in quotation marks.
Data from Refs.[8,18,19]

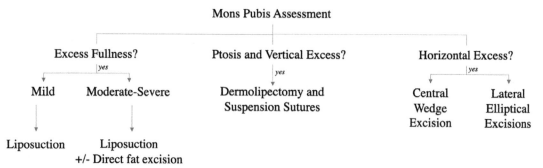

Fig. 1. Suggested assessment and treatment approach to mons pubis deformity.

can preserve deep lymphatics while allowing adequate debulking from the areolar layer to be performed.[4,22] A wedge-shaped segment of fat from the areolar layer can be removed with tissue resection tapered down and limited caudally to the level of symphysis to avoid somatosensory disorders of genitalia.[4,12–15]

In our practice, we use ultrasound-assisted liposuction (VASER, Solta Medical, Bothell, WA) for mons debulking with additional direct fat excision infrequently indicated. Following tumescent liposuction, the subdermal layer is treated with VASER mode (60%–70% power) to achieve skin contracture and tightening, which has been sought after with superficial liposuction and/or lamellar fat excision by other surgeons. The deep fat compartment is treated with the probe on continuous mode (60%–70% power) to allow fat lobule separation and smooth harvest via liposuction cannula while also preserving neurovascular structures and minimizing blood loss.[23] A short 4-mm cannula is optimal for liposuction of the deep fat pocket. Liposuction of the superficial lamellar fat layer is rarely indicated and can result in contour irregularities. When debulking is performed, it is imperative to keep the contour of the pubic region in mind and avoid an unnaturally flattened appearance. The contour over the inguinal region should be flat with mild convexity over the central mons. Liposuction over the inguinal region is minimal, if any, as excess liposuction can result in prolonged edema.

Suspension sutures. In cases of mons ptosis, dermolipectomy alone is insufficient to achieve long-term elevation of the mons. The elevation of the mons must be stabilized with suspension sutures from a strong supporting structure within the mons to a stable point in the lower abdomen and pubis. Scarpa's fascia continues from the abdomen caudally to the level of the labia majora and is continuous with the superficial fascia in the mons. Suspension sutures from the superficial fascia reliably elevate the mons flap. The rectus

sheath acts as a strong anchor point for these suspension sutures. A minimum of 3 suspension sutures are required; additional sutures can be used if further support is required or to eliminate dead space. To avoid neurosensory disturbances, suture placement should be confined from a few centimeters above the anterior commissure to above the pubic symphysis and medial to the external rings.[15] Suspension should be performed to position the anterior vulvar commissure and clitoris at the lower edge of pubis symphysis to avoid undue pull and distortion.[4,9] Care is taken to avoid skin dimpling, irregularities, and an overly pulled appearance of the labia majora. Most surgeons advocate for the use of permanent sutures,[2,4,8,9,14,15,20] whereas others opt for long-lasting resorbable sutures.[12,13] Permanent sutures can help safeguard against ptosis recurrence and may be beneficial in more severe cases of ptosis but present with potential for suture granulomas and abscesses.[4,14]

Alternative approaches to mons suspension have been described but not widely used. El Khatib[8] advocates for dermal-fascial suspension sutures. Following mons liposuction, the skin flap is undermined to the level of suspension sutures. Permanent suspension sutures are then placed from the superficial fascia and dermis of the mons flap to the rectus sheath with intended dimpling. Although El Khatib contends that these dimples soften and fade over time, there is potential for permanent mons contour irregularities that can be difficult to revise and correct. Additionally, a depression between the lower abdomen and mons may be created and intervening fat strangulation and necrosis may occur.[4,9] The superficial fascia of the mons provides sufficient strength for permanent ptosis correction, provided that the superficial layer between the superficial fascia and skin has not been disturbed, which is another reason to avoid fat excision from the superficial lamellar fat layer. Patoue[2] described placing nonabsorbable suspension sutures from the mons to the abdominal fascia centrally and 2 laterally from about 5 cm lateral to the midline of the mons on either side to the ASIS periosteum, with the intent of elevating and spreading their curved dermolipectomy pattern into a straight horizontal line on tension. The authors recognize that the periosteal sutures are painful for up to 15 days postoperatively. Although they note that the pain is transient, long-term dysesthesias from the lateral femoral cutaneous nerve injury, which courses close to the ASIS,[24] can be problematic. In cases of a rounded ptotic mons, the natural delta shape of the mons can be restored with medial-oblique vector of lateral fascial suspension sutures to the rectus fascia to achieve similar goals.[9]

In cases where a concurrent abdominoplasty is performed, the superficial fascia of the mons flap and Scarpa's fascia of the abdominal flap can be anchored to the rectus fascia to stabilize scar position and avoid superior migration.[9] In our practice, we stabilize the abdominoplasty flap separately with an anchor suture from Scarpa's fascia at the midline caudal edge of the abdominal flap to the deep fascia directly overlying the upper pubis symphysis, in addition to progressive tension sutures and Scarpa's layer closure. Anchoring suture of the abdominal flap is placed first before fascial-rectus sheath suspension of the mons as described above.

Horizontal excess correction. Following massive weight loss, the mons skin envelope can also stretch horizontally and require reduction. Mild horizontal excess of the monsplasty incision can be distributed along the abdominoplasty scar, which may result in some early pleating of tissues that settle over time.[13] More significant horizontal excess may require additional skin excision. There are 2 approaches to horizontal skin reduction: a central V-shaped wedge resection[8,9,25,26] or lateral crescentic resections.[1,13,27] The central V-shaped wedge resection is designed as a triangle with the base along the abdominoplasty scar and apex toward the commissure. Drawbacks of this technique include potential for T-junction dehiscence, possible dog-ears near commissure and clitoral hood that can be difficult to revise, central concave deformity of the mons, and risk of clitoral neuropraxia and dyspareunia.[9,13,27] If a vertical wedge resection is considered, we recommend using it in addition to the other monsplasty techniques for debulking, superior dermolipectomy, and suspension, such as El Khatib[8] and not as the sole approach to monsplasty.[25,26] In the latter, incision is more likely to encroach close to vulvar commissure as well as result in central grooving.[9]

Loeb[1] combined monsplasty and upper thigh lift using lateral dermolipectomy. Using the 60°-mons angle as a goal, lateral crescentic incisions were planned on each side from the ASIS to above the subgluteal folds. Same amount of skin was taken above and below the inguinal and crural creases to stabilize the incision. The amount of skin taken above the inguinoabdominal lines varied based on mons deformity (range 3–7 cm). Inferiorly, skin excisions were parallel to labia majora and equidistant from labia majora and respective crural fold. Skin excision was partial; the rest of the undermined lateral flap was deepithelialized and sutured to the deep dermis in the inguinoabdominal region to strength and stability. Similar principles and approach can be used for horizontal mons skin reduction laterally without a concurrent thigh lift. When using lateral excision, suspension sutures are required to prevent lateral and inferior migration of scar, and prolonged edema may be expected.[13] Advantages of this approach include preserved domal mons contour, hair pattern, avoidance of T-junction scars (and "+" junction with concurrent Fleur-de-Lis abdominoplasty), and minimal risk of clitoral deformity and sensory issues.[13,27]

Postoperative Care

In cases of significant fat resection or liposuction and/or dead space formation, a suction drain can be placed to minimize fluid collection. Patients are placed in compression garments for 4 to 6 weeks postoperatively. Heavy lifting and vigorous activity is avoided for the first 6 weeks.

Clinical Outcomes

Restoration of a normal-appearing and positioned mons via monsplasty results in significant quality of life improvements including aesthetic satisfaction, movement, clothing, hygiene, physical exercise, sexual performance, and urinary dysfunction.[8,9,11,12,19] The mechanism of urinary function improvement is not well known but postulated that suspension of the superficial fascia of the mons, which is continuous with Colle's fascia also resuspends and tightens the urogenital triangle.[12]

Complications

When monsplasty is combined with other body contouring procedures, typical complications related to the larger procedures (eg, deep vein thrombosis (DVT)) may occur. In postbariatric patients who undergo monsplasty as part of lower body lift procedures, certain risk factors have been demonstrated to increase the overall risk of complications, including body mass index (BMI) before surgery, highest lifetime BMI, percentage of excess weight, and smoking.[28] Smoking cessation and optimizing healthy diet and lifestyle can help reduce risk of complications.

Bleeding and hematoma. Large vessels can be encountered in the lower abdomen and mons during abdominoplasty and monsplasty. In massive weight loss patients, vessels tend to be enlarged. When monsplasty is combined with abdominoplasty, there is a large contiguous potential space in which hematomas can accumulate. Exact hemostasis with electrocautery and/or ligation with sutures or clips should be performed.

Prolonged edema. Following monsplasty and/or liposuction, prolonged edema common, observed in as much as 70% of patients.[4,9] Mons swelling is expected with gravity-dependent caudal accumulation of edema, especially when monsplasty is combined with larger procedures. As in abdominoplasty, preservation of a thin layer of tissue over the deep fascia (rectus sheath in the abdomen, the Gallaudet fascia in the pubic region) can preserve deep lymphatics while allowing adequate debulking to be performed. Duration and extent of edema can be lessened with use of lymphatic massage, compression garments, cool compresses, and intermittent nondependent positioning of the pelvis (if positioning is not restricted by other concomitant procedures performed).[9,11] Further steps including the elimination of dead space, use of drains as needed, compression garment, and avoidance of shearing movements can help to diminish seroma formation.[22,29] Seromas or lymphoceles are infrequent and can be treated with drainage and compressive dressings.[19]

Infection. Utilization of nonabsorbable sutures for suspension of the mons is recommended by many surgeons to decreases ptosis recurrence.[2] Nonabsorbable sutures, however, may lead to suture granulomas and abscesses that require outpatient treatment.[4,14]

Undercorrection. Undercorrection of the mons typically results from inadequate assessment and treatment planning. When the mons is neglected during body contouring procedures, patients can present with exaggerated fullness of the pubic region, highlighted without coverage of an overlying pannus and against a newly flattened abdomen. Most surgeons plan their inferior abdominoplasty incision at about 6 to 7 cm above the anterior vulvar commissure, which can remove excess vertical skin of the mons. However, if a ptotic mons is not firmly resuspended to its proper position with fascial suspension sutures, correction can be short-lived, and ptosis can recur.[8]

Overcorrection. Overcorrection of mons deformity can result in challenging postoperative issues that can be difficult to revise. Excessive fat resection can create an unnaturally flattened appearance of the mons or pubic concavity. Denuding subcutaneous fat over fascial planes can affect lymphatic drainage, leading to prolonged edema. Overresection of the superior mons skin causes exaggerated elevation of the commissure and anterior rotation of the vulva, which can lead to distortion of the clitoral hood, change in clitoral position and dyspareunia. Additionally, displacement of the urethral meatus can change the angle of urinary stream.[9,15,20] Aggressive reduction of horizontal skin can also affect contour and healing patterns. Midline vertical patterns that encroach on the anterior commissure can potentially create dog-ear deformity near the cleft and placement of a scar in a highly sensitized location. Lateral monsplasty skin excision, if performed aggressively, can flatten out the mons pubis and stretch it horizontally affecting contour, escutcheon, wound healing, and scar migration in an already high-tension location.[19]

Change in pubic hair pattern. One of the criticisms of vertical pull on the mons is that the hair-bearing portion can translocate superiorly and give an elongated appearance to the mons.[26] Horizontal skin reduction through lateral oblique scars can also cause lateral migration of the hair pattern. Patients should be notified of possible changes to escutcheon in advance, which can be addressed later with epilation or laser hair removal.

Genital sensory issues. Sensory innervation of the clitoris can be protected by limiting tissue dissection and resection to the level of the pubic symphysis and not lower, where the nerves can course superficially.[4] Exposure and overstimulation of the clitoris can occur with excessive vertical pull and anterior/superior displacement of the commissure and clitoral hood. Securing the mons such that the anterior commissure is just over the lower pubic symphysis can ensure proper positioning and protect against vertical migration in either direction.

CLINICS CARE POINTS

- Mons deformity should be assessed for 3 parameters to guide surgical planning: excess fatty fullness, ptosis, and the presence of horizontal skin excess in addition to vertical laxity.

- Moderate-to-severe mons ptosis requires suspension of the superficial fascia to the rectus sheath for long-term correction; skin excision alone will likely lead to recurrent ptosis.
- To avoid excess pull on the commissure and vulva, mons suspension should aim to restore the anterior commissure to the lower edge of the pubic symphysis.
- To avoid somatosensory issues, tissue resection from the mons should not be performed caudal to the pubic symphysis.
- Meticulous hemostasis is essential to avoid large hematomas.

ACKNOWLEDGMENTS

The author would like to acknowledge and thank my partner Dr Julie Khanna for her original contributions to surgical techniques described herein as "in our practice."

REFERENCES

1. Loeb R. Narrowing of the mons pubis during thigh lifts. Ann Plast Surg 1979;2(4):290–7.
2. Patoué A, De Runz A, Carloni R, et al. Safe monsplasty technique. J Plast Surg Hand Surg 2018; 52(2):74–9.
3. Yavagal S, de Farias TF, Medina CA, et al. Normal vulvovaginal, perineal, and pelvic anatomy with reconstructive considerations. Semin Plast Surg 2011;25(2):121–9.
4. Kitzinger HB, Lumenta DB, Schrögendorfer KF, et al. Using superficial fascial system suspension for the management of the mons pubis after massive weight loss. Ann Plast Surg 2014;73(5):578–82.
5. Payne R. Chapter 11 - surgical exposure for the nerves of the back. In: Tubbs RS, Rizk E, Shoja MM, et al, editors. Nerves and nerve injuries. London: Academic Press; 2015. p. 155–67. https://doi.org/10.1016/B978-0-12-802653-3.00060-9.
6. Pieroh P, Li ZL, Kawata S, et al. The arterial blood supply of the symphysis pubis - Spatial orientated and highly variable. Ann Anat 2021;234:151649.
7. Tourani SS, Taylor GI, Ashton MW. Scarpa fascia preservation in abdominoplasty: does it preserve the lymphatics? Plast Reconstr Surg 2015;136(2): 258–62.
8. El-Khatib HA. Mons pubis ptosis: classification and strategy for treatment. Aesthetic Plast Surg 2011; 35(1):24–30.
9. Marques M, Modolin M, Cintra W, et al. Monsplasty for women after massive weight loss. Aesthetic Plast Surg 2012;36(3):511–6.
10. Placik OJ, Devgan LL. Female genital and vaginal plastic surgery: an overview. Plast Reconstr Surg 2019;144(2):284e–97e.
11. Furnas HJ, Canales FL, Pedreira RA, et al. The safe practice of female genital plastic surgery. Plast Reconstr Surg Glob Open 2021;9(7):e3660.
12. Bykowski MR, Rubin JP, Gusenoff JA. The impact of abdominal contouring with monsplasty on sexual function and urogenital distress in women following massive weight loss. Aesthet Surg J 2017;37(1): 63–70.
13. Bloom JM, Gusenoff JA. Response to "Going in the wrong direction with monsplasty. Aesthet Surg J 2013;33(8):1211.
14. Michaels J, Friedman T, Coon D, et al. Mons rejuvenation in the massive weight loss patient using superficial fascial system suspension. Plast Reconstr Surg 2010;126(1):45e–6e.
15. Alter GJ. Management of the mons pubis and labia majora in the massive weight loss patient. Aesthet Surg J 2009;29(5):432–42.
16. Brower JP, Rubin JP. Abdominoplasty after massive weight loss. Clin Plast Surg 2020;47(3):389–96.
17. Rezak KM, Borud LJ. Integration of the vertical medial thigh lift and monsplasty: the double-triangle technique. Plast Reconstr Surg 2010; 126(3):153e–4e.
18. Song AY, Jean RD, Hurwitz DJ, et al. A classification of contour deformities after bariatric weight loss: the Pittsburgh Rating Scale. Plast Reconstr Surg 2005; 116(5):1535–44 [discussion: 1545-6].
19. Pechevy L, Gourari A, Carloni R, et al. Monsplasty after massive weight loss: assessment of its aesthetic and functional impact. Ann Chir Plast Esthet 2016;61(1):e21–35.
20. Seitz IA, Wu C, Retzlaff K, et al. Measurements and aesthetics of the mons pubis in normal weight females. Plast Reconstr Surg 2010;126(1):46e–8e.
21. Alter GJ. Pubic contouring after massive weight loss in men and women: correction of hidden penis, mons ptosis, and labia majora enlargement. Plast Reconstr Surg 2012;130(4):936–47.
22. Razzano S, Gathura EW, Sassoon EM, et al. Scarpa fascia preservation in abdominoplasty: does it preserve the lymphatics? Plast Reconstr Surg 2016; 137(5):898e–9e.
23. Khanna JJ, Saheb-Al-Zamani M. Enhanced lipocontouring of the arms. In: Ducan D, editor. Enhanced liposuction - new perspectives and techniques. London: IntechOpen; 2021. https://doi.org/10.5772/intechopen.98807.
24. Ducic I, Zakaria HM, Felder JM 3rd, et al. Abdominoplasty-related nerve injuries: systematic review and treatment options. Aesthet Surg J 2014;34(2): 284–97.
25. Filho JM, Belerique M, Franco D, et al. Dermolipectomy of the pubic area associated with

abdominoplasty. Aesthetic Plast Surg 2007;31(1): 12–5. https://doi.org/10.1007/s00266-006-0102-z.

26. Davison SP, Labove G. Going in the wrong direction with monsplasty. Aesthet Surg J 2013;33(8):1208–9.

27. Alter GJ. Response to "Going in the wrong direction with monsplasty. Aesthet Surg J 2013;33(8):1210.

28. Poodt IG, van Dijk MM, Klein S, et al. Complications of lower body lift surgery in postbariatric patients. Plast Reconstr Surg Glob Open 2016;4(9):e1030.

29. Tourani SS, Taylor GI, Ashton MW. Reply: Scarpa fascia preservation in abdominoplasty: does it preserve the lymphatics? Plast Reconstr Surg 2016; 137(5):899e–900e.

Labia Majora Reduction (Majoraplasty)

Maryam Saheb-Al-Zamani, MA, MD, FRCSC*

KEYWORDS

- Labia majora reduction • Majoraplasty • Labiapexy • Liposuction

KEY POINTS

- Labia majora are paired cutaneous fatty folds that contribute to the aesthetics of the external genitalia and the protective coverage of labia minora, clitoris, urethra, and vaginal opening.
- Aging, weight fluctuation, hormonal changes, and saddle activities can alter labia majora shape. Labia majora aesthetics involves evaluation of fatty fullness, skin excess, and tissue laxity.
- Depending on presentation, majoraplasty may involve volume correction through augmentation or debulking and skin laxity/excess improvement using energy-based devices or dermolipectomy.
- Labia majora skin excision should be performed conservatively and with patient in full abduction to avoid a gaping introitus, with the scar placed on the medial border of labia majora.
- Clitoral sensory disturbance can be avoided by limiting tissue excision to lateral to the clitoral hood and pubic symphysis, and superficial to the ischium.

INTRODUCTION

The mons pubis, labia majora, and labia minora constitute the external female genitalia. Although substantial literature has been dedicated to aesthetic surgery of labia minora, labia majora aesthetics are often overlooked. This article aims to familiarize the reader with relevant anatomy, common aesthetic concerns, as well as a well-rounded overview of described approaches to labia majora reduction (majoraplasty). Complications and clinical pearls are discussed to help surgeons avoid potential pitfalls.

Labia Majora Anatomy

Labia majora are paired cutaneous fatty folds that border vulvar cleft laterally. They merge anteriorly to form the anterior commissure at the inferior-most extent of the mons pubis and meet with labia minora posteriorly to form the posterior commissure. The labia majora provide coverage over the labia minora, clitoris, urethra, vaginal opening, and vulvar vestibules and glands.[1]

Dominant blood supply to the external genitalia is provided by the internal pudendal artery, a branch of the internal iliac artery. The internal pudendal artery gives rise to the dorsal artery of the clitoris and the posterior labial artery and the perineal artery, which supply labia minora and majora. Additional supply is from the superficial external pudendal artery, a branch of the femoral artery.[1-4] Venous drainage of the external genitalia occurs via the external and internal pudendal veins toward the femoral and internal iliac veins, respectively.[4]

The labia majora are innervated anteriorly by the ilioinguinal nerve and the genital branch of the genitofemoral nerve. Innervation to the posterior labia majora and clitoris is provided by branches of the pudendal nerve. The pudendal nerve bifurcates at the superficial transverse perineal muscle into superficial and deep perineal nerves, which become the posterior labial nerve and the dorsal nerve of the clitoris, respectively.[1-3] It is important to recognize that the dorsal nerve of the clitoris courses relatively superficially, just deep to the thin tissues over the clitoris.[2]

Financial Disclosures/Conflicts of Interest: None.
Private Practice, ICLS Plastic Surgery, 1344 Cornwall Road, Oakville, Ontario L6J 7W5, Canada
* Corresponding author.
E-mail address: Maryam.s.zamani@gmail.com

plasticsurgery.theclinics.com

Aesthetic Goals and Treatment Indications

Youthful labia majora are full, smooth, wide anteriorly, narrow posteriorly, and measure approximately 9.3 cm in length.[1,3,5] On standing view, labia majora nearly meet in the midline to form the anterior vulvar commissure.[3] In supine position and slight leg opening, the labia majora cover the vaginal opening with minimal labia minora show.[6]

Labia majora are inferior continuations of, and anatomically contiguous with, the mons. Frequently, mons ptosis results in posterior rotation of the labia majora and perceived excess.[3] Primary changes in labia majora can also occur from tissue laxity and excess. Weight gain can lead to fat accumulation and enlargement of labia majora, which can persist despite weight loss. Estrogen influence during puberty and lack thereof with aging affects the size and appearance of female external genitalia. Typically, high estrogen levels cause the mons pubis, labia majora, and labia minora to become thicker and larger. Conversely, depletion of estrogen with aging can result in atrophy of these structures and sagging appearance.[4] Additionally, labia majora enlargement can arise from prolonged saddle pressure, such as in professional cyclists, leading to vulvar lymphadenopathy.[7] A case report of labia majora enlargement from HIV lipodystrophy secondary to chronic antiretroviral therapy has also been described.[8]

Assessment

Patients with labia majora fullness and/or skin excess can present with aesthetic concerns and difficulty in tight-forming clothes, bathing suits, and underwear.[3] Sexual function can be compromised due to excess labia majora fullness and associated depth of vagina. Hygiene can be difficult to maintain leading to chronic fungal infections.[9]

Physical examination and photographic documentation should be performed in standing and lithotomy positions. If there is mons fullness and/or ptosis, elevation of the mons with a monsplasty should be simulated because this also elevates labia majora and allows for the assessment of majora in isolation. When standing, inferior labial protrusion and apparent length of intervulvar cleft is assessed: the intervulvar cleft can be elongated, akin to a "closed clamshell" anteriorly or a "porpoise nose" laterally.[3] If the patient is noted to have labia minora hypertrophy, this must be discussed preoperatively because minora excess will be exaggerated with reduction of labia majora. Patients should be additionally evaluated for pelvic organ prolapse, which can confound the external genitalia appearance. In standing position, the perineum is located on average within 2 cm of ischial tuberosities. If perineum lies below this level at rest or with a Valsalva maneuver, then referral to gynecologist for pelvic organ prolapse evaluation is indicated.[7]

The patient is then evaluated in the lithotomy position to evaluate excess fatty fullness and labial skin laxity and excess. Labia majora excess can present as full prominent majora at one extreme and deflated with skin excess at other extreme. Labia majora tissue excess and labial deflation must be distinguished for proper treatment. Younger patients and/or those with weight gain tend to present with full fatty labia majora that may swell with arousal.[3] Enlarged full labia majora can be treated with debulking, with or without skin excision as indicated by tissue excess or laxity. Perimenopausal women, in contrast, tend to present with labia majora laxity and perceived skin excess, with sagging skin and posterior wrinkling when supine. In order to restore smooth full labia majora, these patients are typically best served with restoration of volume to the labia majora, with fat grafting or filler, and correction of excess lax skin with excision or radiofrequency (RF) skin tightening depending on the degree of deformity.[3] In patients who undergo massive weight loss, the amount of skin laxity and redundancy is typically too significant for less invasive treatment approaches. Skin excision, with or without subcutaneous fat removal, is indicated for the proper treatment of labia majora enlargement in massive weight loss patients. To determine amount of skin that can be safely excised, patients are examined with maximal leg abduction, simulated well in the frog leg position.[10]

Approach

There are currently no well-described classification systems for assessment and treatment of labia majora deformity. A simple algorithm for the treatment of labia majora enlargement that assesses fatty fullness, skin excess, and tissue laxity is proposed in **Fig. 1**.

Labia majora debulking

Mild fullness of the labia majora with skin excess or ptosis can be treated with liposuction alone with expected modest improvement. In order to avoid contour irregularities and bleeding issues, liposuction with small diameter cannulas (3 mm or smaller) should be performed in a superficial plane.[1,7,10,11,12] Improvement with liposuction alone may be inadequate and should be reserved for mild cases only. More effective bulk reduction can be achieved through direct labia majora approach.[8,9,12]

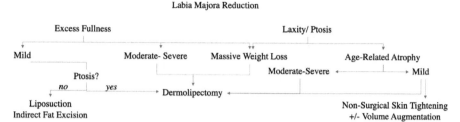

Fig. 1. Suggested assessment and treatment approach for labia majora reduction.

Labia majora skin excision (dermolipectomy)

Widely accepted incision placement for labia majora reduction is on the medial border of labia majora, just lateral to the junction of the hair-bearing labia majora skin and smooth skin of the interlabial sulcus.[1,3,7,9,10,12,13] This scar placement, while being inconspicuous, prevents translocation of hair-bearing skin medially which can be a cause of irritation and dyspareunia.[3]

Conservative tissue excision is planned using a pinch technique in a crescentic pattern from anterior to posterior labia majora. Minimal labia majora tissue excision can be performed continuously in one segment.[3] If more significant removal of tissue is indicated, a more conservative approach involving the elevation of labia majora skin flap from medial to lateral to confirm the amount of redundancy to be removed before committing to the lateral incision line is recommended.[3,7] As much as 50% of the labia majora skin may require excision[3,7] but minimum of 1.5 to 2 cm of labia majora skin laterally should be conserved.[10] Infrequently, in order to avoid a dog-ear deformity at the time of closure, additional tissue may need to be excised through lateral extension anteriorly or posteriorly.[9,10] Incisions should not meet in midline to avoid concentric scar contracture and genital deformity.

If there is excess labia majora bulk, direct excision of superficial fat can be performed at this time. In order to prevent injury to the clitoris, resection should be conservative and lateral to the pubic symphysis and clitoral hood and superficial to the ischium.[10] Meticulous hemostasis with electrocautery needs to be ensured because there are large blood vessels in labia majora and significant hematomas can occur.[3] If significant fat volume is removed, closed-suction drains are placed. Layered closure of Colle's fascia, deep dermis, and subcuticular layer with resorbable sutures is performed.

Majoraplasty combined with other procedures

Labia majoraplasty can be performed in isolation or in combination with other procedures. Some patients become aware of labia majora excess after correction of labia minora hypertrophy.[3,14] Others, present with labia majora and minora hypertrophy concurrently. If simultaneous reduction of labia majora and minora is undertaken, labia majora are reduced first.[12,13]

Labia majora enlargement may also be addressed along with a mons pubis lift.[2,9,10,11] If direct excision of labia majora is not planned, excess bulk may be reduced from the pubic lift incision via liposuction or indirect fat excision. If labia majora excision is to be performed with mons pubic lift, the latter is performed first as labia majora are elevated with raising of the mons. Caution must be exercised in cases requiring monsplasty and majoraplasty if a medial thigh lift has been previously performed because the blood supply to the skin between thighplasty incision and majoraplasty incision may be tenuous. Although majora debulking from the monsplasty incision may be performed, it is recommended to delay skin excision from labia majora to a later procedure.[10]

Finally, labia majora excision may be performed as part of a medial thigh lift[1] or at a separate stage. In order to avoid gaping introitus from lateral tension of medial thigh lifts, labia majora skin excision should be kept conservative.[10]

Postoperative Care

During the first week postoperatively, patients are to pat dry gently after voiding, avoid wiping, and apply antibiotic ointment to the incisions. Sitz baths for short durations can assist with hygiene but prolonged sitting in a hot bath can cause unnecessary vasodilation and edema. Oozing and drainage may be expected initially and pads can be used as necessary. For comfort and to help minimize edema, cool packs applied intermittently to the surgical site are encouraged without direct skin. Patients should wear loose-fitting cotton clothing postoperatively. Regardless of procedure, patients are encouraged to ambulate postoperatively to reduce the risk of deep venous thrombosis. Other light and low impact activities may be resumed within 2 weeks postoperatively. Any heavy lifting (typically more than 10 lbs) and vigorous activities must be avoided for 6 weeks postoperatively. Intercourse and insertion of tampons should be avoided for 6 weeks postoperatively. Patients should avoid positions that place pressure on the perineum such cycling or horseback riding for a minimum of 6 to 8 weeks.[7]

Outcome

As with other aesthetic genital procedure, labia majora reduction has been associated with improved psychosocial well-being, form, and function. Majoraplasty allows for the reduction of fullness and skin excess, shortening the intervulvar cleft and restoring a more youthful appearance. Patient satisfaction is high and sensation to external genitals can be well-preserved.[3,6,8,13,15]

Complications

Due to the rich vascular anatomy of labia majora and its functional significance in providing cushioning and coverage of other external and internal genital structures, labia majoraplasty is associated with significant potential complications. Awareness of these adverse sequelae is key to avoiding pitfalls and achieving successful surgical outcomes.

Bleeding and hematoma
The vessels encountered during labia majora excision tend to be larger and can retract deep into the fatty tissue.[3,12] Meticulous hemostasis with electrocautery is essential as large hematomas can occur. Hematomas must be treated promptly in the operating room under general anesthesia for proper evacuation and source control. Placement of a drain may be indicated.

Prolonged edema
Due to the dependent position of the labia majora, edema and swelling are expected sequelae of surgery. Excision of tissues should be performed superficially to avoid disturbance of the lymphatic drainage network. Edema may be more pronounced with liposuction than with superficial tissue excision.[12] If majoraplasty is combined with monsplasty, fat excision should be conservative and sufficient tissues should be kept to maintain lymphatics; otherwise, significant prolonged edema of not only the mons and labia majora but also of labia minora and clitoral hood can ensure.[9] Professional cyclists should be advised in advance that vulvar lymphadenopathy may limit long-term results.[7]

Poor scarring
Relative to labia minora reduction, labia majoraplasty carries a higher risk of scar hypertrophy.[3] Depending on the location, labia majora skin has different characteristics: it is smooth and hairless along the interlabial sulcus and has coarse pilosity centrally. As the labia majora are followed laterally, pilous density is reduced, the skin is thinner, and increased lateral tension is encountered with leg abduction.

Incision location plays a significant role in scar outcome. Mottura[6] published one of the first descriptions of labia majora reduction, using lateral incisions placed 1 cm medial to crural creases. Lateral scars can be conspicuous and lead to wound dehiscence and even worse, potential gaping of the introitus from high tension and lateral pull on the labia.[1] Lapalorcia[8] described treatment of labia majora HIV lipodystrophy with scar placement in the midportion of the labia majora, with medial and lateral incisions at least 1.5 cm from the medial labial edge and crural crease, respectively. Although hair growth may conceal a central scar, ingrown hairs and cyst formations are potential issues as is flattening or indentation of the caudal labia majora. Optimal location for labia majoraplasty scar placement, rather, is on the medial border of the labia majora, just lateral to the hair-bearing border. This scar placement allows for concealment, minimal tension, and avoids translocation of hair bearing skin into the smooth interlabial sulcus.[1,3,7,9,10,12,13]

The amount of tissue resection can also affect scar outcome. Overresection of labia majora can cause scar hypertrophy and excess visibility from flattening of the labia majora and undue tension on the scar.[3] Labia majora excision should be performed with pinch assessment of the tissue excess with legs in full abduction to ensure minimal pull on the healing incision site. Resection of skin can be assessed with D'assumpcao clamps or incrementally with coronal slits made to assess skin flap width before sagittal excision of the excess skin.

Overresection
Labia majora reduction should be performed to restore the labia majora to their normal form and function. Sufficient labial fat must be maintained to preserve adequate cushioning during intercourse and with saddle activities, such as cycling. Overresection of labia majora can result in a flattening deformity, and worse, a gaping introitus. The latter is a disastrous and difficult-to-correct complication that can lead to vaginal dryness, irritation, and discomfort in clothes. Additionally, overresection can limit leg abduction resulting in

activity limitation, sexual dysfunction, and emotional distress.[7,10]

Sensory disorders

Sensation to the clitoris can be protected by limiting fat excision from the mons to superior to the pubic symphysis and from the labia majora to lateral to the pubic symphysis and clitoral hood and superficial to the ischium.[10]

Future Directions

Energy-based skin-tightening devices have been developed for the improvement of skin laxity in lieu of, or synergistic with, excisional surgery.[16] Dermis and subcutaneous heating to 60°C to 80°C and skin surface to 40°C induces skin tightening via dual mechanisms: initial cleavage of collagen fibril hydrogen bonds and fibrospetal shrinkage followed by neocollagenesis, angiogenesis, and elastin reorganization through the wound healing cascade.[17] Thus far, most of the literature on energy-based skin tightening has focused on body contouring and facial rejuvenation thus far, with sparse attention to external genital applications.

Studies on vaginal rejuvenation and improving stress urinary incontinence and orgasmic dysfunction with RF energy (Thermiva, Themi, Irving, TX) applied to the vagina and external genitalia (labia majora, labia minor, mons, perineal body, clitoral hood, and clitoris) have indirectly depicted improved labia majora laxity.[3,18,19] Recently, Dayan and colleagues[20] published a 10-patient case series on aesthetic and functional improvement of labia majora and minora with RF (Accutite, InMode, Lake Forest, CA). Reported patient satisfaction was high and all were willing to repeat the procedure again. Tightening of the clitoral hood, introitus, forchette, and improved distribution of darkly pigmented labia minora was described by the treating surgeon, and patient recovery was expedited with return to physical and sexual activities by 14 days. Dayan did not include any indicators of labia majora laxity but the clinical example published demonstrated improved mild-to-moderate majora laxity. Introduction of RF-based technologies that specifically aim to improve external genitalia laxity through superficial (eg, Thermiva; Votiva, InMode), transcutaneous microneedling (Morpheus 8V, InMode), and subdermal (Aviva, InMode) applicators, can provide a minimally invasive treatment gap for mild labia majora skin laxity. Potential benefits of RF treatment of labia include avoiding scarring and associated scalloping/irregularities, flap necrosis, hematoma, and overresection of traditional excisional approaches. Future studies focused on labia majora improvement with RF are needed to support clinical efficacy and safety.

SUMMARY

The mons pubis and labia majora are often neglected aesthetic units. Thorough assessment of the mons as part of body contouring and of labia majora as part of external genitalia rejuvenation is central to proper treatment planning and harmonious surgical outcomes. These procedures can be performed safely and effectively and yield high patient satisfaction.

CLINICS CARE POINTS

- Labia majora should be assessed for fatty bulkiness, tissue laxity, and excess skin.
- Isolated mild labia majora fatty fullness can be treated with liposuction. More notable majora enlargement necessitates direct dermolipectomy.
- Perimenopausal women with atrophy and mild skin excess can be treated with volume restoration and energy-based skin tightening. More notable skin excess and/or laxity associated with massive weight loss require skin excision.
- Labia majora skin excision should be conservative and planned with patient in full abduction to avoid a gaping introitus.
- Optimal scar placement is on the medial border of the labia majora, just lateral to the hair-bearing skin, which is inconspicuous and preserves the smooth hairless interlabial sulcus.
- In order to avoid clitoral sensory disturbances, labia majora tissue excision should be kept superficial, lateral to the clitoral hood and pubic symphysis, and superficial to the ischium.
- Meticulous hemostasis is essential to avoid large hematomas.

REFERENCES

1. Triana L, Robledo AM. Refreshing labioplasty techniques for plastic surgeons. Aesthet Plast Surg 2012;36(5):1078–86.
2. Placik OJ, Devgan LL. Female genital and vaginal plastic surgery: an overview. Plast Reconstr Surg 2019;144(2):284e–97e.

3. Hamori CA. Aesthetic surgery of the female genitalia: labiaplasty and beyond. Plast Reconstr Surg 2014;134(4):661–73.

4. Nguyen JD, Duong H. Anatomy: abdomen and pelvis, female external genitalia. In: StatPearls. Treasure Island (FL): StatPearls Publishing; 2021. Available at: https://www.ncbi.nlm.nih.gov/books/NBK547703/.

5. Lloyd J, Crouch NS, Minto CL, et al. Female genital appearance: "Normality" unfolds. BJOG 2005;112:643–6.

6. Mottura AA. Labia majora hypertrophy. Aesthet Plast Surg 2009;33(6):859–63.

7. Furnas HJ, Canales FL, Pedreira RA, et al. The safe practice of female genital plastic surgery. Plast Reconstr Surg Glob Open 2021;9(7):e3660.

8. Lapalorcia LM, Podda S, Campiglio G, et al. Labia majora labioplasty in HIV-related vaginal lipodystrophy: technique description and literature review. Aesthet Plast Surg 2013;37(4):711–4.

9. Alter GJ. Pubic contouring after massive weight loss in men and women: correction of hidden penis, mons ptosis, and labia majora enlargement. Plast Reconstr Surg 2012;130(4):936–47.

10. Alter GJ. Management of the mons pubis and labia majora in the massive weight loss patient. Aesthet Surg J 2009;29(5):432–42.

11. Felicio Yde A. Labial surgery. Aesthet Surg J 2007; 27(3):322–8.

12. Hunter JG. Labia minora, labia majora, and clitoral hood alteration: experience-based recommendations. Aesthet Surg J 2016;36(1):71–9.

13. Miklos JR, Moore RD. Simultaneous labia minora and majora reduction: a case report. J Minim Invasive Gynecol 2011;18(3):378–80.

14. Di Saia JP. An unusual staged labial rejuvenation. J Sex Med 2008;5(5):1263–7.

15. Ostrzenski A. Labiopexy and labioplasty for labium majus rejuvenation in light of a newly discovered anatomic structure. Aesthet Plast Surg 2014;38(3):554–60.

16. Khanna JJ, Saheb-Al-Zamani M. Enhanced lipocontouring of the arms. In: Ducan D, editor. Enhanced liposuction - New perspectives and techniques. London: IntechOpen; 2021. https://doi.org/10.5772/intechopen.98807.

17. Theodorou SJ, Del Vecchio D, Chia CT. Soft tissue contraction in body contouring with radiofrequency-assisted liposuction: a treatment gap solution. Aesthet Surg J 2018;38(Suppl 2):S74–83.

18. Magon N, Alinsod R. ThermiVa: the revolutionary technology for vulvovaginal rejuvenation and noninvasive management of female sui. J Obstet Gynaecol India 2016;66(4):300–2.

19. Alinsod RM. Transcutaneous temperature controlled radiofrequency for orgasmic dysfunction. Lasers Surg Med 2016;48(7):641–5 [Erratum in: Lasers Surg Med. 2017;49(7):727].

20. Dayan E, Ramirez H, Theodorou S. Radiofrequency treatment of labia minora and majora: a minimally invasive approach to vulva restoration. Plast Reconstr Surg Glob Open 2020;8(4):e2418.

Female Sexual Dysfunction

Michael A. Reed, MD

KEYWORDS

• Female sexual dysfunction • Low desire • Orgasm disorder • Sexual pain • GSM

KEY POINTS

- Persistent, distressful, recurrent problems with sexual arousal, desire, orgasm, and/or sexual pain make up the disorders ascribed to female sexual dysfunction.
- Causes of diminished interest and arousal can stem from disruptions in life, partnership issues, hormonal issues, and/or medical conditions and associated treatments.
- Psychotherapy, directed masturbation training, and sensate focus are the three primary treatment pathways for orgasmic disorders.
- Genitourinary syndrome of menopause (GSM) represents only one example of sexual pain disorders in women. Lubricants, moisturizers, and hormonal and nonhormonal treatments exist for the treatment of GSM.
- It is important for the clinician to be able to distinguish the difference between a "dysfunction" and a "dissatisfaction."

INTRODUCTION

Female sexual dysfunction (FSD) is an umbrella term encompassing several facets of sexuality in terms of desire, arousal, orgasm, and/or sexual pain. Persistent, recurrent problems with sexual arousal, desire, orgasm, or pain that distress the patient or strain the relationship with their partner are known medically as sexual dysfunction. Many women experience problems with sexual function at some point in their lives, and it is estimated that in the United States 40% of women have sexual complaints.[1] FSD can occur at any stage of life and can drastically curtail quality of life for many women. It can occur only in certain sexual situations or in all sexual situations. These conditions are often underdiagnosed and undertreated despite sexual health being a necessary component of general medical care throughout the life cycle of women. Given the high prevalence of FSD, it is reasonable that all physicians, surgeons, and health care professionals have basic education and tools available to guide patients and assist clinicians in reaching a diagnosis and treatment strategy. Patient evaluation begins by understanding the different *Definitions of Female Sexual Dysfunction*.

1. *Female sexual interest/arousal disorder (FSIAD)* replaces the Diagnostic and Statistical Manual of Mental Disorders (DSM) IVs hypoactive sexual desire disorder (HSDD) and arousal disorder, which were listed as separate conditions but are now combined as FSIAD in DSM V. This revised classification has been controversial among experts in the area of sexual medicine because there is little empirical support or validation of the new diagnostic category/criteria in contemporary clinical research (for the purpose of this article. FSIAD and HSDD will be used interchangeably). The DSM V defines FSIAD as the absence or significantly reduced sexual interest/arousal for at least 6 months (with at least three of the following symptoms): (a) absent/reduced interest in sexual activity, (b) absent/reduced sexual/erotic thoughts or fantasies, (c) no/reduced initiation of sexual activity; unresponsive to partner's attempt to initiate sexual activity, (d) absent/reduced sexual excitement/pleasure during

The author has no financial disclosure or conflicts of interest with presented material in this article.
4627 Fermi Place Suite 110, Davis, CA 95618, USA
E-mail address: drreed@drmichaelreed.com

Clin Plastic Surg 49 (2022) 495–504
https://doi.org/10.1016/j.cps.2022.06.009

sexual activity in at least 75% of encounters, (e) absent/reduced sexual interest/arousal in response to any internal or external cues (eg, written, verbal, visual), (f) absent/reduced genital or nongenital sensations during sexual activity in at least 75% of sexual encounters.[2]

2. *Orgasmic disorder* is defined as the absence, delay, infrequency, or marked diminishment in intensity of orgasm in at least 75% of sexual experiences, persisting for at least 6 months and causing distress.[3]

3. *Sexual pain disorders* can involve any part of the female anatomy. Whether the disorder involves the vulva, vagina, cervix, uterus, adnexa, or the pelvic floor muscles, the common thread is sexual pain. The three most frequently used terms to describe sexual pain disorders in women are: vulvodynia, dyspareunia, and vaginismus. This article focuses on dyspareunia, and the most common cause of dyspareunia in a postmenopausal woman is genitourinary syndrome of menopause (GSM).

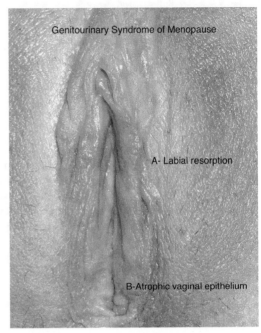

Fig. 1. GSM.

PATIENT EVALUATION

Given the high prevalence of FSD, it is reasonable that all physicians, surgeons, and health care professionals have basic education and tools available to guide patients and to assist clinicians to reach a diagnosis and treatment strategy.

Initial consultation with a patient regarding sexual dysfunction should begin with a specialized tool, having the patient self-report regarding sexual function by completing a validated questionnaire such as the Female Sexual Function Index (FSFI-6) **(Fig. 1)**. Over the past 20 years, the FSFI has been considered the gold standard for the measurement of sexual function in women.[4] The FSFI-6 is a 6-item self-report covering five components of sexual function: arousal, satisfaction, desire, pain, and lubrication. By having the patient complete an FSFI-6, you are given a window into the patient's overall level of sexual function as well as the primary components that are causing her sexual dysfunction.

As health care professionals, it is our responsibility to take a patient-centered, nonjudgmental, and mutual respect approach when discussing sexual dysfunction with our patients. It begins in the privacy of an office with the patient dressed and by providing an environment that is comfortable, relaxing, and establishes mutual trust. Patients often appreciate it if you, as a provider, acknowledge the difficulty they might be experiencing when discussing the sexual realities of their life. Encourage the patient to list their "bothers" followed by a list of the patient's own "goals" on completion of her treatment.

Understanding her "bothers" allows you, as the provider, to begin to have an idea of the distress, and potential causes, as well as working as a Segway to tease more essential information from the patient to reach a diagnosis. Some suggested interview questions that can assist with eliciting more information are:

1. How long have you been dealing with this problem in your life?
2. How often do you have sexual thoughts or fantasies?
3. Is your sexual life fine or good, fair, or unsatisfactory?
4. Do you have any problems with vaginal dryness, vulvar pain, or irritation?
5. Does your partner have sexual or erectile issues?
6. Do you have any present or past situations of verbal, physical, or sexual abuse?
7. What are you hoping to achieve from treatment?

Asking open-ended questions gives your patient "permission" to include sexual issues as part of her presentation, and gives you, the clinician, a window into her surgical rationale and sexual health.

Diminished Interest and Arousal (Female Sexual Interest/Arousal Disorder) in Women

1. *Causes:*
   a. *Disruptions of life:* Disruptions can come in many forms, including: new demands from work as she is climbing the ladder, dealing

with bureaucracy, experiencing perimenopausal symptoms of irregular bleeding, night time hot flashes, exhaustion after a recent childbirth or being the primary provider for young children to name just a few.

b. *Partnership issues:* This heading could be expansive albeit but includes such as martial issues, financial stressors, and partner's difficulty in achieving or maintaining his erection.

c. *Hormonal issues:* This can be either estrogen or testosterone-related or both. If estrogen related, many women may experience irregular, unpredictable bleeding, hot flashes, vaginal dryness, or have difficulty sleeping. Experiencing these symptoms is not conducive to improving arousal or interest. Ovaries produce estrogen, but they also contribute testosterone. Testosterone helps with memory and increases motivation, self-confidence, and heightens interest in sex. Diminishing testosterone levels can be seen in postmenopausal women as well as in younger women on oral contraceptives, frequently resulting in adverse effects on interest and arousal.

d. *Medical conditions and their associated treatments:* Any medical condition that interrupts the activities of daily living will adversely affect sexual response as it relates to interest and arousal. The most common conditions related to our discussion are depression, hypertension, diabetes, heart disease, and cancer. Many treatments for these common conditions are a double-edged sword and can diminish sexual interest and arousal. Frequently implicated are antidepressant medications such as tricyclics (Elavil), selective serotonin reuptake inhibitors (Prozac and Zoloft), antihypertensive agents (Inderal and Procardia), and sedatives (Xanax and Valium).

2. *Therapy:* The first step for the practitioner is to accurately identify what is going on with the patient. Is the patient's lack of interest and arousal associated only with her libido? Are there other factors affecting her interest and arousal, such as problems of inadequate vaginal lubrication, pain, and orgasmic dysfunction? (This will be discussed later. in this article.) The FSFI 6 is a validated questionnaire and an excellent short form to use in the office to help understand other possible causes related to diminished interest and arousal. Therapy for diminished interest and arousal (FSIAD) in women usually follows one or more of the four separate pathways of treatment:

a. *Easing perimenopausal/menopausal symptoms* and relieving insomnia. Initiating hormone replacement therapy (HRT) to optimize her hormonal milieu to alleviate hot flashes, night sweats, mood alterations, and insomnia can definitely revitalize one's interest and arousal.

b. *Relieving vaginal dryness/burning* and improving her ability to lubricate can have a life-altering effect when it comes to intimacy, connection, interest, and arousal. For more specific recommendations of treatment, see Genitourinary Syndrome of Menopause section, which is discussed later in this article.

c. *Psychotherapy* focusing on modifying thoughts, beliefs, behaviors, and emotions by using any of the following cognitive approaches: the permission, limited information, specific suggestions, intensive therapy (PLISSIT) model, sensate focus, cognitive behavior therapy, and mindfulness-based therapy.

d. *Medications* included in the treatment of FSIAD include flibanserin, bremelanotide, testosterone supplementation, and bupropion.

    i. Flibanserin is a nonhormonal multifunctional serotonin agonist and antagonist that results in a decrease in serotonin activity and an increase in dopamine and norepinephrine activity.[5] Daily dosing of flibanserin 100 mg at bedtime has demonstrated increased sexual desire, decreased sexually related distress, and increased satisfying sexual events.[6] The most common adverse events in premenopausal women were dizziness (9.2%), somnolence (8.3%), nausea (6.5%), and fatigue (3.7%). Most of these symptoms can be mitigated by bedtime dosing. Flibanserin has a boxed warning that highlights the increased risks of "serious hypotension and syncope" with concomitant use of alcohol. It is generally recommended that if the patient consumes more than two mixed drinks or the equivalent, the evening dose should not be taken nor should the patient double the dosage in the morning. Efficacy may not emerge for several weeks, and treatment should be discontinued after 8 weeks if no benefit is realized.[7]

    ii. Bremelanotide is an on-demand subcutaneous autoinjection given 45 minutes before sexual activity. Melanocortins have been associated with excitatory pathways in the brain and linked to appetitive sexual behaviors.[8] Bremelanotide is an analog of alpha-melanocyte-stimulating hormone with high affinity for the melanocortin-4 receptor, resulting in modulation of neurotransmitter pathways involved in sexual desire and arousal in women with HSDD. This modulation demonstrates a significant improvement in desire and a decrease in distress related to a lack of desire.

The most common adverse effects include nausea (39.9%), facial flushing (20.4%), and headache (11%). Prescribing guidelines recommend no more than one dose in 24 hours and no more than eight doses per month.[9]

iii. Testosterone therapy is an evidence-based, off-label treatment most commonly for perimenopausal and postmenopausal women with FSIAD.[10] In double-blind, placebo-controlled clinical trials in naturally and surgically menopausal women, testosterone therapy resulted in statistically significant improvements in the number of satisfying sexual events, sexual desire, and improvement in prior sexual distress twofold greater than placebo. Testosterone is best administered, intramuscularly or transdermally via a patch, cream, or pellet. Orally administered testosterone results in a significant rise in the amounts of low-density lipoprotein (LDL) cholesterol and reductions in total cholesterol, high-density lipoprotein (HDL), and triglycerides. The administration of testosterone by way of cream, pellet, or patch is preferred because of its neutral effects on lipid profile.[11] The most common adverse events include hirsutism and acne. Efficacy may not emerge for several weeks, and treatment should not be continued beyond 6 months if no benefit is realized.

iv. Bupropion is antidepressant that works as a norepinephrine-dopamine reuptake inhibitor that has been used off-label to improve decreased sexual desire. Despite multiple adverse effects such as tremor (13.5%), agitation (9.7%), dry mouth (9.2%), constipation (8.7%), excessive sweating (7.7%), dizziness (6.1%), and nausea/vomiting (4%) when given sustained-released 150 to 400 mg daily has been investigated in several clinical trials for treatment of FSIAD.[12,13]

Orgasmic Disorder is a dysfunction disorder that effects as many as 42% of women at some time during their lifespan. Female orgasmic disorder is characterized by a significant change in orgasm such as delay, reduction of intensity, or cessation. "Orgasm" may be defined as a buildup of pleasurable sensations and excitement to a peak intensity that releases tension and creates a feeling of satisfaction and relaxation.[1]

Orgasms may be classified as clitoral or vaginally activated. Clitoral orgasms are usually more commonly achieved and are the result of direct manual stimulation of the visible portion of the clitoris with either one's own finger, a partner's body part, or a toy; they may additionally be achieved via sexual fantasy. Vaginally activated orgasms are thought to be caused by the internal stimulation of the bulbs and crus of the clitoris, and the autonomic supply to Grafenberg's Area by massaging the anterior vaginal wall, digitally, via penile–vaginal intercourse, or with a sexual toy. Vaginally activated orgasms are less common and experienced by ~30% of women.[14] It is important to reassure the patient that an "orgasm is an orgasm" whether it is clitoral or vaginally achieved.

The female sexual response of desire, excitement, plateau, orgasm, and resolution in a linear fashion as first ascribed by Masters and Johnson, in 1966, is inaccurate when describing female sexual response. First described in 2000 by Dr Rosemary Basson, current thinking involves a circular model, incorporating the importance of emotional intimacy, sexual stimuli, and relationship satisfaction. The circle is a pleasure oriented, not a goal-oriented model, where any activity can lead to pleasure, and there is not a goal of orgasm.[1] The goal is personal satisfaction, which can manifest as physical satisfaction (could be orgasm) and or emotional satisfaction (intimacy with a partner). This is especially important when counseling patients who are expecting a certain outcome from their sexual engagement.

Causes: Self-image, societal norms, cultural beliefs, and even myths can shape our feeling of normalcy or sense of dysfunction when addressing thoughts and beliefs about sexuality. As physicians, we have an obligation to correct misinformation that could be perpetuating a patient's distress. Common myths that perpetuate orgasmic dysfunction include:

1. If a woman does not experience orgasms through vaginal intercourse, there must be something wrong with her.

2. If a woman is unable to experience an orgasm with a partner but has no problem experiencing one through masturbation, it will mean that her partner is not a compatible one.
3. Lesbian women are attracted to women because they have never experienced "real pleasure" with a man.
4. Female orgasms are given to women by their partners.

Therapy in women usually follows one or more of the three separate pathways of treatment:

1. *Sensate focus* is a sex therapy technique introduced by Masters and Johnson, whereby the participants refocus on their own sensory perceptions and sensuality instead of goal-oriented behavior focused on the genitals and penetrative sex. The aim is to minimize pressure and expectations and to appreciate new sensual possibilities.
2. *Directed masturbation training* consists of weekly therapy and masturbatory exercises to be practiced by the patient. This includes visual examination of the vulva and whole body, with exploration and touching. Each session increases the intensity of exploration and touching along with supplementing fantasy and erotica. It is reported that this technique is extremely effective, resulting in 90% of women becoming orgasmic during treatment.[1]
3. *Psychotherapy* remains the mainstay treatment for orgasmic disorders and has been shown to be effective in helping women to gain or regain the ability to have orgasms. Given the multidimensional nature of orgasmic disorder, it is extremely important to have an effective, accessible, and expert network for referral and support.

SEXUAL PAIN DISORDERS
Vulvodynia

Chronic unexplained pain involving the vulva for greater than 3 months is by definition *vulvodynia.* This pain disorder usually involves severe pain at the vaginal entrance which can be elicited by a number of activities including vaginal pressure from intercourse as well as nonsexual activities like tampon insertion or bicycle riding. The typical descriptors given by patients include but are not limited to burning, cutting, sharp, and searing pain of the vaginal opening. Often times the examining physician may not find any observable cause of the pain. Despite the lack of clinical findings, the patient's experience of pain should be validated.

The diagnosis and treatment of vulvodynia is complex and requires the physician to rule in/out known causes of vulvar pain such as infection (eg, yeast vulvovaginitis) or dermatologic disease (eg, lichen sclerosis) of the vulva. If a diagnosis of a known cause of vulvar pain is made, then the patient does not have vulvodynia. If the health care provider is unable to make a diagnosis of a known cause of vulvar pain, then the patient is diagnosed with vulvodynia.[15]

The typical treatments for vulvodynia start with noninvasive treatments such as psychological interventions, pelvic floor physical therapy, or alternative treatments such as acupuncture and hypnosis.[16] Depending on the patient's progress, treatments may progress to include medical treatments.

Neuromusculoskeletal problems can cause or contribute to chronic pelvic and sexual pain disorders in many women. Overactive pelvic floor muscles, specifically the puborectalis, levator ani, pubococcygeus, and the musculature of the introitus can result in pain in the posterior vestibule. This condition of overactive pelvic floor muscles is referred to as *vaginismus*.

Clinically, vaginismus makes sexual intercourse difficult or impossible, secondary to involuntary contractions of the vaginal muscles.

Pelvic floor *physiotherapy* under the direction of a pelvic floor physical therapist aids the patient by developing awareness and control of the vaginal musculature as well as restoring function, improving mobility and relieving pain and overcoming vaginal penetration anxiety.

Pharmacological treatments consist of local anesthetics such as lidocaine, muscle relaxants, neuroleptics, or anxiolytic medications. Local anesthetics are aimed at reducing pain by decreasing discomfort on penetration. This decreased pain also decreases anxiety with resultant diminution of muscle spasms of the pelvic floor. Botulinum toxin, a temporary muscle paralytic, has been recommended in the treatment of vaginismus by decreasing the hypertonicity of the pelvic floor muscles.[17]

Psychological treatments are often based on the notion that vaginismus results from relationship problems, negative sexual experiences in childhood, or a lack of sexual education. Individual therapy may focus on identifying and resolving underlying psychological problems that could be causing the disorder. Cognitive behavioral sex therapy also involves the resolution of underlying causes and may incorporate the use of vaginal dilators as means to desensitize the patient to vaginal penetration.

Vulvodynia is a complex multifactorial pain condition that can result in significant sexual and psychological distress for affected women.

Interventions and resolution of their complaints require an interdisciplinary model of care. The surgeon when encountering this subset of patients should be judicious when considering to perform female cosmetic procedures. These procedures may only worsen her sexual disorder.

Genitourinary Syndrome of Menopause

Historically, GSM was referred to as vulvovaginal atrophy, atrophic vaginitis, or urogenital atrophy. The terminology change was initiated in 2014 by both the North American Menopause Society (NAMS) and the International Society for the Study of Women's Sexual Health (ISSWSH), because these terms were not considered clinically accurate and "atrophy" carries a negative connotation for most women, thus making the terminology GSM more inclusive.[18]

Evaluation

GSM can potentially be diagnosed after listening to the patient's history. It is important during the history to elicit onset, duration, and quality of symptoms, including understanding if/how these symptoms impact their sex life. Physical examination of the vulva and vagina should not be deferred as other vulvar dystrophies can cause similar anatomical changes to the vulva, such as lichen sclerosis (see **Fig. 1; Fig. 2**).

GSM can affect every anatomical structure of the vulva. The changes that are seen are the direct result of decreasing sex steroids, in particular estrogen and testosterone. Associated changes with decreasing levels of estrogen and testosterones can consist of changes to the labia majora, clitoral phimosis, labial resorption, thinning of the vaginal epithelium, vulvar vestibule/introitus, urethra, and bladder as well as an increase in vaginal pH. Increased vaginal pH changes the microbiome resulting in the overgrowth of pathogenic bacteria of the vagina and bladder which can cause symptoms of vaginitis, urinary urgency, stress incontinence, dysuria, and recurrent urinary tract infections. GSM not only affects anatomical structures of the vulva but can have negative effects regarding women's emotional well-being, sexual functioning and relationships, and body image. In the Women's Voices in the Menopause study, 40% of women impacted by GSM reported a negative impact on their sex life. Almost one-third reported the vaginal symptoms made them "feel old." In another study, GSM adversely affected sexual interest, intimacy, and relationship with the partner. Sixty-one percent of women made excuses to avoid intercourse because of their symptoms and feeling less confident.[18]

Treatment options

The goal for treating GSM is to alleviate the most commonly reported symptoms. These symptoms include irritation of the vulva, inadequate vaginal lubrication, burning, dysuria, dyspareunia, and vaginal discharge. Treatment can be accomplished with both pharmacological and non-pharmacological treatments.

Pharmacological Treatments

Vaginal estrogens, estradiol (E2), or estriol (E3) are considered the gold standard for the treatment of GSM. According to NAMS and the International Menopause Society, vaginal estradiol therapy is considered to be the first-line pharmacological treatment.[19] Achieving replete estrogen stores to the tissues results in more dynamic, resilient, and thickened vaginal epithelium. Although vaginal estradiol reduces the symptoms of GSM, the systemic absorption is low and will not alleviate hot flashes or reduce the risk of osteoporosis. Recent studies have not shown an elevated risk of cardiovascular disease, endometrial, breast, ovarian, colorectal cancer, or hip fracture. However, vaginal estradiol is contraindicated in women with undiagnosed abnormal genital bleeding.

The typical dosing for vaginal estradiol is ~10 micrograms daily for 14 days, then twice weekly. This ultra-low-dose vaginal estradiol is as effective as low-dose tablets (25 μg) and more effective than placebo. This treatment regimen

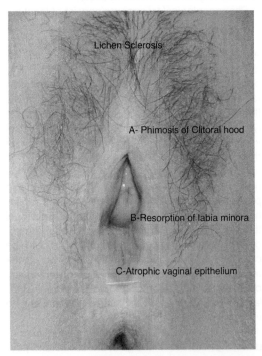

Lichen Sclerosis

A- Phimosis of Clitoral hood

B-Resorption of labia minora

C-Atrophic vaginal epithelium

Fig. 2. Lichen sclerosis.

results in reduction in vaginal pH and improved dyspareunia, vaginal dryness, and urogenital symptoms with minimal safety concerns. Even with ultra-low-dose vaginal estradiol, some systemic absorption will occur. Despite systemic circulating estrogen, there is no evidence of endometrial proliferation or the need for routine ultrasonography.[18] Low-dose vaginal estradiol comes in a variety forms including, but not limited to, vaginal creams, low-dose estradiol vaginal ring, and estradiol vaginal inserts.

Intravaginal Dehydroepiandrosterone (Prasterone)

Dehydroepiandrosterone (DHEA), androstenedione, and testosterone are collectively known as androgens. Androgen receptors are located throughout the genitourinary tract. These structures include the glans clitoris, urethra, minor vestibular glands, and periurethral and vulvar vestibule (introitus). In healthy premenopausal women, androgen production is significantly greater than that of estrogen and is the necessary precursor substrates for biosynthesis of estrogens. Decreasing androgens with advancing age can be a contributory factor in the development of the signs and symptoms of GSM.[20]

Prasterone is a synthetic equivalent to endogenous DHEA and is approved for the treatment of moderate to severe dyspareunia. Prasterone is an inactive precursor that is converted locally into estrogens and androgens with minimal systemic exposure. Intrarosa does not carry a boxed warning on its label and has no restrictions on duration of use but has not been tested in women with breast cancer or history of breast cancer. Prasterone is administered as a 6.5 mg vaginal insert once daily at bedtime[21] or may be compounded usually as a 10 mg cream or suppository dosage. With daily use, patients can expect improvement in sexual function by improving vaginal dryness, decreasing pH as well as improvements in urogenital symptoms. Minimal safety concerns exist regarding the usage of DHEA for the treatment of GSM. Large randomized controlled studies have shown endometrial safety in both short- and long-term trials.[18] The most common side effect of prasterone is vaginal discharge, and it is contraindicated in women with undiagnosed abnormal genital bleeding.

Selective Estrogen Receptor Modulators (Ospemifene/Osphena)

SERMs are drugs that act like estrogens on some tissues but block the effect of estrogen on other tissues. Osphena is the first and only selective estrogen receptor modulator (SERM) taken once-daily, orally. It is a nonhormonal treatment of moderate to severe vaginal dryness and/or moderate to severe painful intercourse, symptoms of changes in and around the vagina due to menopause.[22]

Nonhormonal Treatments: Lubricants and Moisturizers

Nonhormonal treatments are not definitive cures, but work to temporarily relieve the signs and symptoms of GSM. The anatomical changes associated with this syndrome as discussed before will continue to progress in the background while using these remedies.

Lubricants are designed to minimize friction and irritation during intercourse around the clitoris, labia, and vaginal entrance. It is recommended that both partners apply lubricant to their genitals to decrease pain, but also add pleasure, comfort, and increased ease of orgasm. Different formulations of lubricants exist and are generally categorized as water-based, oil-based, or silicone-based. Each of these categories of lubricants has their own particular advantages and disadvantages. Water-based lubricants include Sutil, Unbound Jelly (flavored lube), Good Clean Love (best for sensitivities), astroglide, and many others. Water-based lubricants are the best option for people with sensitivities, particularly when no parabens, propylene glycol, or additives are present. They are typically odorless, do not decrease the efficacy of condoms, and can be used with all sex toys, including those composed of silicone. Being composed mostly of water, these lubricants tend to absorb quickly and can often leave the patient feeling dry and tacky, which will require multiple applications during intercourse. Hence, water-based lubricants are not recommended for anal sex, extra passionate playtime, or activities in the shower, bathtub, or pool. Oil-based lubricants such as olive oil, coconut oil, or a light "pleasure oil" are not as easily absorbed and tend to provide longer sustained relief from friction, irritation, and discomfort during intercourse. Oil-based lubricants tend to be a bit messy and can break down latex condoms, decreasing the efficacy of this type of contraceptive method. Last, oil-based lubricants can increase the frequency of vaginal infections in those patients that are troubled by easily recurring vaginitis. Silicone-based lubricants such as Uberlube and Sliquid Naturals Silver provide long-lasting comfort without the need to reapply. Silicone is compatible with latex condoms and is the preferred lubricant for anal sex.

Moisturizers are designed to increase vaginal moisture by rehydrating the dry mucosal tissues. They adhere to the vaginal lining and mimic natural vaginal secretions by binding to water. They can be applied anytime and are meant to be used on a consistent basis over a longer period of time in hopes to help with the day-to-day feelings of dryness and scratchiness. When recommending vaginal moisturizers, the products recommended should help maintain the proper pH and osmolality of the vagina.

Non-pharmacological treatments

Energy-based treatments are generally classified as either radio frequency, laser (fractional CO2, Yag), or high-intensity focused ultrasound. These treatments use different forms of energy to accomplish the similar results by remodeling collagen and elastin and improving blood flow via neovasculogenesis. These treatments seem to be safe and effective with minimal downtime. The improvements in sexual function have been in the areas of desire, arousal, lubrication, orgasm, satisfaction, and pain.

Relieving systemic menopausal symptoms

Many patients who suffer from GSM often times will have systemic symptoms of menopause. Vasomotor symptoms are the most commonly reported, but vaginal dryness, painful intercourse, adverse mood, poor sleep, and cognitive complaints all seem to worsen as women approach menopause.[23] These complaints can be mitigated if not adjudicated by prescribing systemic HRT. Unfortunately, the prevailing thought among women and clinicians regarding the risk/benefit perception of HRT continue to remain distorted and its use is avoided. HRT reduces all-cause mortality and risks of coronary disease, osteoporosis, and dementias.[24,25] It is our responsibility as physicians to be able to have a discussion with our patients regarding HRT.

Therapies currently available include oral estrogens, combined oral estrogen and progestin products, transdermal patches, creams, gels, and injectable, for example, pellets. The ideal regimen begins by assessing your patient for comorbid conditions and tailoring dosing to rapidly control symptoms. The safest "window of opportunity" to prescribe HRT is within 10 years after the patient's last menstrual cycle. An example of a usual starting dose is 1 mg oral estradiol or 0.05 mg transdermal estradiol patch. Despite oral estrogens having been prescribed the longest and most researched, the prevailing thought is to avoid orals as they increase the risk of blood clots and or stroke.

To the contrary, transdermal preparations of estradiol whether a patch, cream, gel, or pellet DO NOT increase the risk of blood clots or stroke. Estradiol creams can also be compounded by your local compounding pharmacy to your exact prescribing specifications. If your patient still has her uterus, you will need to prescribe some sort of progesterone or progestin. Micronized progesterone is preferred over synthetics like medroxyprogesterone acetate at a minimum dose of 100 mg nightly.

Moreover, the misinterpretation of research findings, such as the Women's Health Initiative Study (WHI) as it pertains to breast cancer risk continues to generate irrational fear of HRT by both medical professionals and the general population. Most women will not be diagnosed with breast cancer as a result of their exposure to HRT. Of those women only taking unopposed estrogen (hysterectomized women), the risk of associated breast cancer is associated with little to no change in risk. Finally, those women who take combined HRT (estrogen + progesterone) can be associated with a duration-dependent increased risk of breast cancer. Beyond 10 years of use of HRT, the absolute excess risk of developing breast cancer is small, less than 10 additional cases per 1000 women aged 50 to 59.[24] Although the WHI trial does NOT prove that estrogen or estrogen + bioidentical progesterone to be unsafe. It finds that giving estrogen, especially estrogen plus the synthetic progestin medroxyprogesterone, to older women for the purpose of cardio protection and bone loss prevention only is ill-advised and short-sighted. Like most, if not all, pharmacological interventions, insignificant risks may exist. Thus, the potential for minor increase in breast cancer risk after 10 years of HRT should be disclosed and discussed with patients as a standard of care. This patient-centered approach creates transparency and shared decision-making between the patient and the prescriber. Moreover, it allows for informed consent and gives the patient the right to self-determine about risk and benefit of this treatment option for women suffering from menopausal symptoms. For patients who choose to accept this clinical intervention, it is recommended that you meet with them, annually, to review any changes in their medical health and discuss advances in medicine, women's health specifically, to ensure goal-centered individualized GSM and/or menopausal treatment regimens for each patient.

SUMMARY

Surgeons undertaking female cosmetic surgery should have a basic understanding of the classifications, possible causes, and potential treatment strategies for patients struggling with sexual dysfunction. Dysfunctions are not amenable to surgery and often times only make these disorders worse. Dissatisfaction about one's own body or specifically genitalia is surgically responsive and seems to improve self-image and "satisfaction."[26] As a practicing cosmetic gynecologist caring for women daily, it is imperative that we understand the importance of discerning the difference between dysfunction versus dissatisfaction. By having this understanding, you will be better able to counsel patients as to whether an operation will achieve her desired goal or to make the appropriate diagnosis, treatment, or necessary referral that would better serve the patient than the surgery itself.

CLINICS CARE POINTS

- Diminishing testosterone levels can be seen in postmenopausal women as well as in younger women on oral contraceptives, frequently resulting in adverse effects on interest and arousal.

- The administration of testosterone by way of cream, pellet, or patch is preferred because of its neutral effects on lipid profile.

- Botulinum toxin, a temporary muscle paralytic, has been recommended in the treatment of vaginismus by decreasing the hypertonicity of the pelvic floor muscles.

- Genitourinary syndrome of menopause (GSM) can affect every anatomical structure of the vulva; vaginal estrogens, estradiol (E2), or estriol (E3) are considered the gold standard for the treatment of GSM. The typical dosing for vaginal estradiol is ~10 micrograms daily for 14 days, then twice weekly.

- Nonhormonal treatments are not definitive cures, but work to temporarily relieve the signs and symptoms of GSM. Oil-based lubricants can increase the frequency of vaginal infections in those patients that are troubled by easily recurring vaginitis.

REFERENCES

1. Goldstein I, Clayton AH, Goldstein AT, et al. Textbook of female sexual function and dysfunction diagnosis and treatment. Chichester, UK: John Wiley & Sons, Ltd; 2018. 198–200, 206–208.

2. American Psychiatric Association. Diagnostic and statistical manual of mental disorders. 5th ed. Washington, DC: American Psychiatric Association; 2013.

3. Marchand E. Psychological and behavioral treatment of female orgasmic disorder. Sex Med Rev. Published online October 2020. doi:10.1016/j.sxmr.2020.07.007.

4. Rosen R, Brown C, Heiman J, et al. The Female Sexual Function Index (FSFI): a multidimensional self-report instrument for the assessment of female sexual function. J Sex Marital Ther 2000;26:191–208.

5. Filbanserin [prescribing information]. Bridgewater, NJ: Valeant Pharmaceuticals. Available at: http://www.accessdata.fda.gov/drugsatfda_docs/label/2015/022526lbl.pdf. Accessed March 12, 2022.

6. Dimon JA, Kingsberg SA, Shumeil B, et al. Efficacy and safety of filbanserin in postmenopausal women with hypoactive sexual desire disorder: results of the SNOWDROP trial. Menopause 2014;21(6):633–40.

7. Seftel AD. Re: hypoactive sexual desire disorder: international society for the study of women's sexual health (ISSWSH) expert consensus panel review. J Urol 2017;198(2):235.

8. Kingsberg SA, Clayton AH, Portman D, et al. Bremelanotide for the treatment of hypoactive sexual desire disorder. Obstet Gynecol 2019;134(5):899–908.

9. Mayer D, Lynch SE. Bremelanotide: new drug approved for treating hypoactive sexual desire disorder. Ann Pharmacother 2020. https://doi.org/10.1177/1060028019899152.

10. Krapf JM, Simon JA. The role of testosterone in the management of hypoactive sexual desire disorder in postmenopausal women. Maturitas 2009;63(3):213–9.

11. Islam RM, Bell RJ, Green S, et al. Safety and efficacy of testosterone for women: a systematic review and meta-analysis of randomised controlled trial data. Lancet Diabetes Endocrinol 2019. https://doi.org/10.1016/s2213-8587(19)30189-5.

12. Segraves RT, Clayton A, Croft H, et al. Bupropion sustained release for the treatment of hypoactive sexual desire disorder in premenopausal women. J Clin Psychopharmacol 2004;24(3):303–16.

13. Bupropion [prescribing information]. Research Triangle Park, NC: GlaxoSmithKline. Available at: https://www.gsksource.com/pharma/content/dam/GlaxoSmithKline/US/en/Prescribing_Information/Wellbutrin_Tablets/pdf/WELLBUTRIN-TABLETS-PI-MG.PDF.Revised April 2016. Accessed March 12 2022.

14. Goodman MP, Adams D. The midlife bible : a woman's survival guide. Robert D. Reed; 2007. p. 107–9.

15. Bornstein J, Goldstein AT, Stockdale CK, et al. 2015 ISSVD, ISSWSH and IPPS consensus terminology and classification of persistent vulvar pain and vulvodynia. Obstet Gynecol 2016;127(4):745–51.

16. Curran S, Brotto LA, Fisher H, et al. The ACTIV Study: acupuncture treatment in provoked vestibulodynia. J Sex Med 2010;7(2):981–95.

17. Lahaie MA, Boyer SC, Amsel R, et al. Vaginismus: a review of the literature on the classification/diagnosis, etiology and treatment. Women's Health 2010;6(5):705–19.

18. Kagan R, Kellogg-Spadt S, Parish SJ. Practical treatment considerations in the management of genitourinary syndrome of menopause. Drugs & Aging 2019;36(10):897–908.

19. North American Menopause Society. The role of local vaginal estrogen for treatment of vaginal atrophy in postmenopausal women: 2007 position statement of the North American Menopuse Society. Menopause 2007;14(3 pt1):355–69.

20. Simon JA, Goldstein I, Kim NN, et al. The role of androgens in the treatment of genitourinary syndrome of menopause (GSM): International Society for the Study of Women's Sexual Health (ISSWSH) expert consensus panel review. Menopause 2018;25(7): 837–47.

21. AMAG Pharmaceuticals. Introsa (prasterone) vaginal insert. Prescribing information 2018.

22. Duchesnay Inc. Osphena (Ospemifene) tablets: prescribing information. 2019.

23. Langer R, Hodis HN, Lobo RA, et al. Hormone replacement therapy - where are we now? Climacteric 2021;24(1):3–10. https://doi.org/10.1080/13697137.2020.1851183.

24. Marsden Jo, Pedder H. HRT and breast cancer risk – fast facts. Post Reprod Health 2021;27(1):42–4. https://doi.org/10.1177/2053369120973424.

25. Santoro N, Epperson N, Matthews S. Menopausal Symptoms and Their Management. Endocrinol Metab Clin North Am 2015;44(3):497–515. https://doi.org/10.1016/j.ecl.2015.05.001.

26. Goodman MP, Placik OJ, Matlock DL, et al. Evaluation of body image and sexual satisfaction in women undergoing female genital plastic/cosmetic surgery. Aesthet Surg J 2016;36(9):1048–57.

Noninvasive Vulvar and Intravaginal Treatments

Erez Dayan, MD

KEYWORDS

- Noninvasive labiaplasty • Vulvovaginal rejuvenation • Pelvic floor restoration • Radiofrequency

KEY POINTS

- Radiofrequency is an effective and safe method for both pelvic floor restoration and nonsurgical labiaplasty.
- Bipolar radiofrequency with temperature control is more effective than monopolar radiofrequency for volumetric heating of vulvovaginal tissue.
- Combination of electrical muscle stimulation and radiofrequency can provide combined nonsurgical restoration of the vulvovaginal tissues.

INTRODUCTION

Since its first description in the plastic surgery literature in the 1980s labiaplasty and vulvovaginal treatments have rapidly increased in popularity.[1] The American Society of Aesthetic Plastic Surgery reported 12,756 labiaplasty surgeries in 2018, more than a 53% increase over the last 5 years. The growing popularity vulvovaginal procedures have been attributed to decreased stigmatization, changes in fashion trends, and increased exposure to nudity in social media.[2] Over the last 20 years, energy-based devices including radiofrequency and laser (CO2 and Erbium:yttrium-aluminum-garnet [YAG]) have been used successfully in aesthetic and functional procedures.[3] The goal of these energy-based devices have been to contract soft tissue and stimulate neocollagenesis and neoangiogenesis. Indications for these devices included vaginal laxity, dryness, vaginal atrophy, itching, dyspareunia, and urinary incontinence.

Erbium:YAG laser devices emit a wavelength of 2940 nm with a penetration depth of 1 to 3 um of tissue per J/cm^2 allowing for surface injury with minimal thermal damage to surrounding tissue. The mechanism is to contract vulvovaginal mucosa through neocollagenesis. This contraction does not tighten the vaginal tone but rather contracts mucous membranes. Different devices

have developed micropulses combined with long-pulse modes to control the heating of target mucous membranes inside the vaginal canal.[4,5] FotonaSmooth (Dallas, TX, USA), Action II (Goyang, South Korea), and MCL 31 Demablate (Jena, Germany) used in clinical trials have demonstrated decrease in Visual Analogue Scale (VAS) scores of both vaginal dryness and dyspareunia, increase in Vaginal Health Index Score, improvement in spontaneous urinary incontinence, improvement in postvoid residual urine volume, and improvement in International Consultation on Incontinence Questionnaire-Urinary Incontinence scores. Histologic findings suggested better elasticity of the vaginal wall with tightening and firming. Adverse events were mild and included transient edema and tolerable heating sensation and rare spotting.[6–9]

Numerous carbon dioxide lasers have been developed for vulvovaginal restoration (FemiLift, SmratXide [Florence, Italy], MonaLisa Touch [Florence, Italy], AcuPulse [Yokneam, Israel], Co2RE Intima [Wayland, MA, USA]). The CO2 laser ablates tissue by emitting light at a wavelength of 10,600 nm, targeting water in tissue. Carbon dioxide is 20X less specific than Erbium, which develops more heat spread to surrounding tissues, leading to neocollagenesis and alteration of vaginal mucosa. Numerous studies have shown improvement in ICIQ-UI, reduction in vaginal

Avance Plastic Surgery, 5588 Longley Lane, Reno/Tahoe, NV 89511, USA
E-mail address: DrDayan@avanceinstitute.com

Clin Plastic Surg 49 (2022) 505–508
https://doi.org/10.1016/j.cps.2022.07.004

dryness, improvement in dyspareunia, improvement in VAS scores for all symptom categories, and improvement of VHI scores. Adverse events reports have been limited to mild discomfort, swelling, and mild bleeding.[10–12]

This article focuses on radiofrequency, which more recently has emerged as a promising minimally invasive treatment for both treatment of the labia as well as pelvic floor. Radiofrequency (RF) is a familiar technology in most fields of medicine (ie, orthopedics, cardiology, oncology, etc.). Its first use was in the 1920s for electrocautery.[13] RF consists of an electromagnetic current that is applied through tissue (ie, skin, muscle, collagen). RF generates heat as a result of different tissue resistance or impedance to the electromagnetic current; this follows Ohm's law: Energy (J) = Current^2 x Resistance x Time.[14] For example, collagen has a higher tissue impedance than muscle and will preferentially generate more heat for a given amount of time.[15] For example, when RF energy is directed to the subdermal adipose tissue, it has been shown to generate temperatures 7X higher than those generated by the dermis, leaving to fat necrosis with epidermal preservation.[16]

Modern minimally invasive and noninvasive radiofrequency devices have shown promise in vulvovaginal restoration. Over the past 10 years, radiofrequency devices have advanced to deliver RF in a bipolar fashion (vs monopolar) with continuous temperature control, both elements that are important to controlled volumetric heating over the duration of treatment.[17] Early monopolar radiofrequency devices delivered energy to tissue with the electrical current moving toward a remote grounding pad. Many of these devices lacked temperature control or measured tissue surface temperature as a surrogate for internal temperature, which led to treatments that were either underpowered or reached temperatures in an uncontrolled fashion, increasing the risks of complications such as burn injuries. The use of bipolar radiofrequency avoids the need for a remote grounding pad and thus allows for volumetric heating of tissue.[18] The bipolar devices use continuous internal and external temperature monitoring, which have significantly improved the safety and efficacy of vulvovaginal RF treatments.

DISCUSSION

In our practice, both minimally invasive and noninvasive bipolar radiofrequency devices are used for treatment of the vulvovaginal region. Laxity of the vulvovaginal tissue can occur for a variety of reasons, including natural aging, childbirth, genetics, and trauma. These events can lead to generalized symptoms such as stress urinary incontinence, atrophic vaginitis, dyspareunia, or aesthetic dissatisfaction. Stress urinary incontinence is a prevalent problem affecting up to 35% of all adult women.[3] Further, an estimated 76% of women have symptoms of sexual dysfunction that significantly affect their quality of life.[19,20]

Treatment of the Labia Majora and Minora

Both labia majora and minora are treated with a combination of minimally invasive bipolar radiofrequency (Aviva, InMode Lake Forest, CA, USA) as well as fractional radiofrequency (Morpheus, InMode, Lake Forest CA, USA)[21,22] (**Figs. 1** and **2**). These procedures both can be performed comfortably under local anesthesia. First, a detailed medial history and physical is obtained including patient expectations. The distance from midline to free edge of the labia minor when extended laterally is measured to assess pretreatment and posttreatment labia hypertrophy. Labia minora hypertrophy is determined at a distance of greater than 5 cm. Patients are typically premedicated with 10 mg of oral diazepam and 5/325 mg of hydrocodone with acetaminophen. One dose of oral antibiotics is given preoperatively (cephalexin or ciprofloxacin). The patient is standardly prepped and draped and placed in stirrups. Access points at the caudal aspect of the labia minora and majora on each side are injected with 3 to 5 cc of 1% lidocaine with epinephrine. Next a 14-gauge needle is used to create a puncture site for access. A 20-gauge spinal needle is then used to infiltrate 20 to 40 cc of tumescent solution (50 cc of 2% lidocaine, 12 cc sodium bicarbonate, 1.5 mg epinephrine per liter of lactate ringers) per treatment site. Water-soluble ultrasound gel is then placed over the treatment areas to allow for bipolar radiofrequency conduction. Next the bipolar radiofrequency internal cannula is placed through the access port with the external electrode on the surface of the labia. The device is activated with target temperatures of 38 C externally and 60 C internally. The device is moved in a craniocaudal motion until the targets reach these target temperatures and maintain them for approximately 30 to 45 seconds. Next the fractional RF device was used to treat the labia majora and minora at depths of 4, 3, and 2 mm and an energy of 20 to 30; this was done in double pulse fashion and 50% overlap of pulses.

In our studies evaluating this treatment, preoperative measurements of labia hypertrophy and protrusion had a mean of 4.4 cm (+/− 1.3) and 3.9 (+/− 2.3) respectively. Measurements at

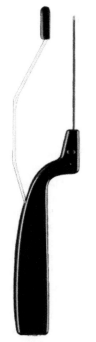

Fig. 1. Bipolar radiofrequency device for soft tissue contraction of labia majora and minora (Aviva). (*Courtesy of* InMode, Lake Forest, CA.)

6 months postprocedure showed an average improvement of 2.7 (+/− 2.2) and 3.1 (+/− 2.3), representing a 38.6% (STD ± 15.3) and 20.5% (STD ± 17.4) change.

Treatment of the Vaginal Canal

In our practice, for internal pelvic floor treatment we use a combination of noninvasive bipolar radiofrequency (Votiva, InMode Lake Forest, CA, USA) and fractional radiofrequency (MorpheusV InMode, Lake Forest, CA, USA) in combination with an internal electrical muscle stimulation device (EmPower Inmode Lake Forest, CA, USA)[21,22] (**Fig 3**). RF applied to the vaginal wall has been shown to stimulate proliferation of glycogen-enriched epithelium, neovascularization, and collagen formation.[4] Once the noninvasive bipolar device reaches temperatures between 40 and 45 C, an inflammatory cascade is initiated and heat shock proteins induce fibroblasts, which leads to neocollagenesis and estogenesis.[4,23] In a previous study that our group conducted with this technology objectively measuring pelvic muscle contraction (Urostym, Portsmouth, NH), there was a direct correlation between treatments and improved pelvic muscle floor contraction. Histologic biopsies of vaginal mucosa at 3 months posttreatment demonstrate increase in elastic fiber density compared with baseline biopsy. The biopsies also find no damage to the submucosal collagen layer and no scar tissue formation in posttreatment, verifying no adverse effect of the fractional RF treatment. Although data are currently being collected to evaluate the objective contribution of electrical muscle stimulation of the pelvic floor, there is evidence of show that a synergy exists.

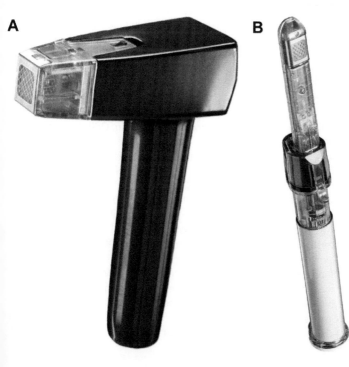

Fig. 2. Fractional radiofrequency device for treatment of labia majora and minors. (*A*) Morpheus8 and (*B*) Morpheus8V. (*Courtesy of* InMode, Lake Forest, CA.)

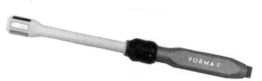

Fig. 3. Internal bipolar radiofrequency device for pelvic floor restoration (Votiva, Lake Forest, CA). (*Courtesy of* InMode, Lake Forest, CA.)

SUMMARY

- The use of bipolar radiofrequency is safe and effective for the treatment of both functional and aesthetic concerns in the vulvovaginal area.
- Temperature control has been the major advance to allow for volumetric heating without complications.
- Combination therapies (ie, addition of electrical muscle stimulation) may prove to be synergistic with radiofrequency for vulvovaginal restoration.

DISCLOSURE

Consultant/Investigator: InMode. Book Royalties: Elsevier, Thieme. Co-Founder: Core Aesthetics LLC.

REFERENCES

1. Mayer HF. Vaginal labiaplasty: current practices and a simplified classification system for labial protrusion. Plast Reconstr Surg 2015;136(5):705e–6e.
2. Goodman MP. Female genital cosmetic and plastic surgery: a review. J Sex Med 2011;8(6):1813–25.
3. Preminger BA, Kurtzman JS, Dayan E. A systematic review of nonsurgical vulvovaginal restoration devices: an evidence-based examination of safety and efficacy. Plast Reconstr Surg 2020;146(5): 552e–64e.
4. Tadir Y, Gaspar A, Lev-Sagie Ahinoam, et al. Light and energy based therapeutics for genitourinary syndrome of menopause: consensus and controversies. Lasers Surg Med 2017;49(2):137–59.
5. Karcher C, Sadick N. Vaginal rejuvenation using energy-based devices. Int J Womens Dermatol 2016;2(3):85–8.
6. Fistonic N, Fistonic I, Gustek S, et al. First assessment of short-term efficacy of Er:YAG laser treatment on stress urinary incontinence in women: prospective cohort study. Climacteric 2015;18(Suppl 1): 37–42.
7. Ogrinc UB, Sencar S, Lenasi H. Novel minimally invasive laser treatment of urinary incontinence in women. Lasers Surg Med 2015;47(9):689–97.
8. Pardo JI, Sola VR, Morales AA. Treatment of female stress urinary incontinence with Erbium-YAG laser in non-ablative mode. Eur J Obstet Gynecol Reprod Biol 2016;204:1–4.
9. Lapii GA, Yakovleva A, Neimark A, et al. Study of proliferative activity of vaginal epithelium in women with stress urinary incontinence treated by Er:YAG laser. Bull Exp Biol Med 2017;163(2):280–3.
10. Athanasiou S, Pitsouni E, Grigoriadis T, et al. Microablative fractional CO2 laser for the genitourinary syndrome of menopause: up to 12-month results. Menopause 2019;26(3):248–55.
11. Samuels JB, Garcia MA. Treatment to external labia and vaginal canal with CO2 laser for symptoms of vulvovaginal atrophy in postmenopausal women. Aesthet Surg J 2019;39(1):83–93.
12. Eder SE. Early effect of fractional CO2 laser treatment in post-menopausal women with vaginal atrophy. Laser Ther 2018;27(1):41–7.
13. Fisher GH, Jacobson L, Bernstein L, et al. Nonablative radiofrequency treatment of facial laxity. Dermatol Surg 2005;31(9 Pt 2):1237–41 [discussion: 1241].
14. Alster TS, Lupton JR. Nonablative cutaneous remodeling using radiofrequency devices. Clin Dermatol 2007;25(5):487–91.
15. Greene RM, Green JB. Skin tightening technologies. Facial Plast Surg 2014;30(1):62–7.
16. Youn A. Nonsurgical face lift. Plast Reconstr Surg 2007;119(6):1951.
17. Dayan E, Burns A, Rohrich R, et al. The use of radiofrequency in aesthetic surgery. Plast Reconstr Surg Glob Open 2020;8(8):e2861.
18. Dayan E, Theodorou S. Not all radiofrequency devices are created equal: a thermal assessment. Plast Reconstr Surg Glob Open 2022;10(2):e4077.
19. Berman JR, Adhikari SP, Goldstein I. Anatomy and physiology of female sexual function and dysfunction: classification, evaluation and treatment options. Eur Urol 2000;38(1):20–9.
20. Berman JR, Berman L, Werbin T, et al. Female sexual dysfunction: anatomy, physiology, evaluation and treatment options. Curr Opin Urol 1999;9(6): 563–8.
21. Dayan E, Ramirez H, Theodorou S. Radiofrequency treatment of labia minora and majora: a minimally invasive approach to vulva restoration. Plast Reconstr Surg Glob Open 2020;8(4):e2418.
22.. Dayan E, Ramirez H, Westfall L, et al. Role of radiofrequency (Votiva, InMode) in pelvic floor restoration. Plast Reconstr Surg Glob Open 2019;7(4): e2203.
23. Qureshi AA, Tenenbaum MM, Myckatyn TM. Nonsurgical vulvovaginal rejuvenation with radiofrequency and laser devices: a literature review and comprehensive update for aesthetic surgeons. Aesthet Surg J 2018;38(3):302–11.

Genital Self-Image and Esthetic Genital Surgery

Sarah A. Applebaum, MD, MS[a,b], Otto J. Placik, MD[a,*]

KEYWORDS

- Female genital self-image • Genital appearance • Esthetic genital surgery • Self-esteem
- Body image • Patient education

KEY POINTS

- The perception of female genital self-image is derived from both psychological and physical etiologies that may be influenced by external influences of idealized standards of beauty and sociocultural norms.
- There is a wide range of what constitutes "normal" genitalia and the general public has a restricted awareness of the extent of normalcy.
- Esthetic genital surgery strives to improve the perception of one's own genital appearance.
- Esthetic genital surgery can have a profound impact on physical distress, psychosexual functioning, and quality of life.
- Patient education and high-quality resources are imperative to changing the stigmatizing landscape of esthetic genital surgery.

BACKGROUND

Definition of Genital Self-Image

Around the world, there is a growing body of literature that has identified an increasing desire to improve one's genital appearance, and it has led to an exponential increase in the number of women seeking esthetic genital surgery each year.[1–4] Although there are a variety of motivations to undergo esthetic genital surgery, the most commonly reported involve appearance.[4,5] Women with a self-perceived "abnormal" genital appearance will seek corrective surgery because their genital self-image is disharmonious with what they perceive to be "normal."[6,7] It has also been shown that women may perceive a "normal" appearance, yet still desire a modification.[1,8]

Much in the same way that patients with body dysmorphic disorder (BDD) are preoccupied with an imagined defect or slight physical anomaly, concern regarding genital appearance has the potential to inflict significant psychosexual distress leading to functional impairments.[6,9] Some have labeled women seeking esthetic genital surgery as having BDD, although BDD may not be all inclusive, as only 18% of women seeking labiaplasty were found to meet diagnostic criteria for BDD in a well-controlled study.[3] Furthermore, unlike esthetic surgery in general, which is rarely beneficial for patients with BDD, as most report unsatisfactory surgical outcomes and maintenance of dysmorphic symptoms postoperatively, most of the patients (95%) undergoing esthetic genital surgery are very appreciative of their outcomes and are generally in agreement that surgery drastically improved the quality of their life.[6,8,10–16] Thus, researchers have proposed that either the validated tool to diagnose BDD (Yale-Brown Obsessive-Compulsive Scale) is not capable of detecting symptoms of dysmorphia related to genital appearance, or the conventional thinking that BDD will not improve after surgery may need to be modified when genitalia are involved.[17,18]

[a] Division of Plastic Surgery, Northwestern University Feinberg School of Medicine, 880 West Central Road, Street 6100, Arlington Heights, IL 60005, USA; [b] Department of Surgery, University of Maryland Medical Center, 22 South Greene Street, S8B02, Baltimore, MD 21201, USA
* Corresponding author.
E-mail addresses: sappleb2@gmail.com (S.A.A.); otto@bodysculptor.com (O.J.P.)

Clin Plastic Surg 49 (2022) 509–516
https://doi.org/10.1016/j.cps.2022.06.004
0094-1298/22/© 2022 Elsevier Inc. All rights reserved.

History of Genital Self-Image

The evolution of female genital self-image may best be understood in terms of the history of esthetic genital surgery. Although the topic has gained increased media attention over the last 20 years, the first documented labiaplasty was performed in 1978 when a 19-year-old woman underwent "50% resection" of the labia minora.[19] Since then, physicians have developed procedures in genital modification to address physical complaints, targeting both esthetic and functional concerns.[17] However, in doing so, public prejudice and controversies in the medical community regarding extremes of size, symmetry, and global perceptions and expectations of the female form have culminated in strong stigmatizing opinions of women undergoing esthetic genital surgery.[20]

Scrutiny surrounding a patient's motivation for modification has driven both patients and physicians alike to define and overemphasize physical differences as an indication for surgery.[8,20] However, in the literature, mixed data regarding normal labial width are pervasive, with reports ranging from 3 mm to 50 mm in an adult patient.[21] As such, there is no clear definition of labial hypertrophy and cutoff values to justify surgery should generally be avoided.[21–23] Others have attempted to reevaluate labia size in terms of subjective perception of size and self-reported complaints. In a cross-sectional study of 200 patients, the objective size of one's labia was found to be significantly associated with subjective perception; however, there was no significant influence of size on self-reported complaints.[22] Although women may be cognizant of their own variations in anatomy, this awareness in and of itself does not necessarily shape one's sense of self nor does it motivate one to seek surgical intervention.

A lack of consensus on the definition and significance of labia size has led others to justify esthetic genital surgery in terms of "sexual function," postulating that attitudes toward genital appearance may be related to dyspareunia (physical pain during sex) or "sexual dysfunction" (nonphysical inability to become aroused or achieve an orgasm).[24] However, this hypothesis fails to account for the fact that a history of vulvodynia, dyspareunia, or chronic pelvic pain is relative contraindications to vaginoplasty, which has been criticized for increasing intercourse-related pain.[25,26] A recent cross-sectional study of 196 women undergoing esthetic genital surgery (including 64% vaginoplasty, 47% labiaplasty, 13% filler augmentation of labia majora, 10% labia majora reduction, and 3% liposuction plus fat transfer) reported intercourse-related pain as "rare or never" in 97% of patients before surgery, yet in 38% of patients after surgery, representing a 59% increase in the number of women reporting intercourse-related pain because of surgery.[14]

In relation to "sexual function", preoperative and postoperative functioning is typically reported as a broad term that encompasses both physical pain and arousal depending on its definition. This makes it hard to draw meaningful conclusions from studies that report a change as well as to compare results between studies. Moreover, data pertaining to sexual function are often collected through patient surveys, adding another layer of complexity to the interpretation of significant findings. Because men and women can have "wet dreams," we believe that "sexual function" as it relates to one's ability to become aroused and achieve an orgasm is largely supratentorial in nature and therefore inextricably intertwined with genital self-image.[27] Although we are not going to address sexual function in and of itself, it is impossible to separate the two. Thus, taken together, there is a need to define genital self-image as being strictly an "esthetic" preference—without relating it to anatomy, medical conditions, or sexual function.

Factors that Influence Genital Self-Image

Social media

Since its inception in 1996, more than half of the world's population has become engaged with social media;[28] 84% of its users are less than 29 year old and 78% are of the female sex.[29] Although the first social media platforms were created to facilitate networking and engagement with family and friends, they now provide instantaneous and continuous access to informational, educational, and cultural resources across the globe. Owing to its accessibility, 43% of users of age 25 to 40 years reported using social media as its daily news source in 2021.[30]

In light of these statistics, the powerful impact of the media on what constitutes cultural norms and expectations cannot be overstated. It should not come as a surprise that information pertaining to genital appearance is not readily available in modern day life, and thus the media serves as the only avenue to access more obscure content for most individuals.[20,31] In women seeking esthetic genital surgery, the vast majority were introduced to surgery through the media.[1,24] In addition, media exposure to beauty ideals has been found to be the greatest predictor of whether or not a woman would seek labiaplasty.[1,24,32] In a well-controlled study of 35 women considering labiaplasty, a greater exposure to media images was not only identified among women who underwent surgery, but also the strength of their desire for surgery was commensurate with the volume of images reviewed.[4]

It turns out that no one is immune to the potentially harmful effects of the media. After viewing images of idealized standards of the female body, body dissatisfaction scores in a sample of college students worsened irrespective of one's body mass index or body dissatisfaction score before the viewing.[33] In another study, the extent of exposure to either modified or non-modified genitalia was found to impact women's perceptions of subsequent images as representing normal or a societal ideal. The group of women exposed to non-modified genitalia was more likely to rate other non-modified images as "normal," and the group exposed to modified genitalia was more likely to rate modified images as "normal." Despite these unsurprising findings, both groups indicated an overall tendency to rate images of modified genitalia as being "more ideal."[34]

Taking the impact of the media one step further, in recent years, the Internet and other technologies have facilitated and normalized access to pornography, with more than half of young adults reporting their first exposure to pornography in adolescence, and 20% feeling unattractive or sexually inadequate as a result of that exposure.[35] Similarly, in women seeking esthetic genital surgery, pornography consumption has been correlated with lower genital self-image and self-esteem.[1] Thus, the media's depiction of female body type frequently informs the general public of societal ideals and, what's more, young women are particularly susceptible to self-criticism in the face of an unrealistic portrayal.[31]

Childbearing

A little less than half of the patients seeking esthetic genital surgery first reported distress about the appearance of their vagina after giving birth.[1] During childbirth, the ligaments, fascia, and other connective tissues around the vagina are physiologically stretched, resulting in a reduction in vaginal tightness and changes in postpartum sexual function, including both physical pain and an inability to orgasm in the absence of pain. Rates of decreased sexual function as high as 86% at 2 to 3 months and 64% at 6 months have been identified in postpartum women.[36–39] A multivariate regression analysis reported changes in body image and genital self-image account for 14.1% of the variance identified in sexual function.[40]

Cultural expectations

Pubic hair A qualitative Internet-based survey study of genital preferences identified pubic hair as the most commonly stated dislike in women

and the second most common in men.[41] Pubic hair removal techniques via shaving, waxing, or lasers are generally expensive and very unpleasant, characterized by skin irritation, ingrown hairs, folliculitis, and rashes, not to mention discomfort with genital exposure.[42] Yet, owing to a strong social drive to uphold its practice, pubic hair removal has been on the rise in younger women, which has likely contributed to an increased awareness of genital tissue that was previously hidden.[35,43]

Male versus female perspectives Regarding male versus female preferences for female genital appearance, men are typically more pleased and positive about the appearance of a woman's genitalia, and negative reactions from a male partner are rarely cited as the motivation for undergoing genital modification.[8,41]

Female genital mutilation/cutting More than 200 million women have experienced female genital mutilation/cutting (FGM/C), a medically unnecessary and often ritualistic, partial or total removal of the external female genitalia.[44] Various communities and cultures have different reasons for practicing FGM/C; however, social acceptance is cited as the most common.[44] Reversal of FGM/C is gaining popularity, although the incidence of this procedure is largely underreported.[45] Most of the women who seek reversal of FGM/C are motivated by a desire to recover their identity, followed by health-related, functional concerns.[46] Postoperatively, most women report feeling satisfied with their outcomes, at least in part, due to improvements in intercourse (less painful, more pleasurable), menstruation, and voiding (50% to 100%).[47–49] Amid the low social acceptance of FGM/C reversal, however, one-third of the patients have been found to prefer the old appearance and perceive their new genitalia to be "abnormal" despite successful reconstruction.[50,51] Compared with health-related, functional concerns, women motivated by identity recovery are typically less likely to be satisfied with their results due to ingrained attitudes from one's upbringing.[49] These results may have implications for women with a history of trauma undergoing genital modification, suggesting the patient's satisfaction with the procedure may be associated with the motivation for surgery.

Trends in Esthetic Genital Image

The emergence of gender fluidity, gender confirmation surgery, and esthetic genital surgery brings into question the concept of "today's esthetics." Beauty has long been the subject of art, culture, and entertainment, and we often alter our appearance and behavior in accordance with the attitudes of society serving as the "gold standard."[31]

Changes in idealized anthropometric prototypes can be appreciated over time. In the twentieth century, trends highlighted popularity of less curvaceous body types to more curvaceous and back to less curvaceous by the end of the century.[52] Now, in the early twenty-first century, we are again seeing a rise in curvaceous body types with soaring rates of the "Brazilian butt lift."[53,54]

A change in paradigm has been observed at the genital level too. Since 1954, *Playboy* centerfold photographs have been serving us depictions of the physically most "attractive" models. Over time, average distance from the horizontal midline of the centerfold photograph to the model's vaginal area decreased, whereas distance from the centerfold to the model's breasts increased, thereby promoting more explicit vaginal content.[55] Pubic hair presentation in these photographs has also transitioned from visibility to invisibility, with trends in the promotion of Brazilian waxing, anal bleaching, and "vajacials" following suit.

In today's world, variations of hair colors, fashion styles, piercings, tattoos, grooming practices, and surgical options are limited only by availability and financial means.[56] Currently, most women seeking esthetic genital surgery express a desire for the smooth, prepubescent "Barbie look."[4,31,36]

As mainstream media and clothing have had an influence on where we are today in terms of an idealized female genital image, we can speculate future projections of genital prototypes that may involve increased ornamentation (will there be a role for genital makeup?). As gender fluidity continues to become more mainstream by promoting body positivity and self-expression, we hope to encounter a similar divergence of esthetic genital image, granting women the freedom and liberty to safely alter their appearance without substantial community and medical backlash.

CLINICAL RELEVANCE
Major Motivators of Esthetic Genital Surgery

The most common motivators of esthetic genital surgery and their incidence have been identified as follows:

1. Esthetic concerns (52.1% to 87%)[1,5,8,57]
2. Physical discomfort when wearing clothes (15% to 64%)[5,57]
3. Low self-esteem, anxiety, or lack of confidence (45.7%)[8]
4. Painful sexual intercourse (43% to 60%)[8,57]

5. Physical discomfort when playing sports (15% to 26%)[5,57]

Benefits and Limitations of Esthetic Genital Surgery

Overall, the literature favorably suggests esthetic genital surgery generates positive patient-reported outcomes, marked improvement in self-esteem, and a significant reduction in symptoms related to the patient's negative genital self-image (including embarrassment, physical discomfort, clothing restriction, and exposure in a bathing suit or other tight garments).[6,58–62] When performed with appropriate training, expertise, and attention to detail in a properly selected patient, esthetic genital surgery is associated with low complication rates between 2% and 13% without long-term sequelae.[13,15,60,63–71]

With respect to limitations, although esthetic genital surgery seems to have a positive effect on self-esteem, most of the studies not only fail to use a validated, quantitative methodology to assess this outcome but also to measure both preoperative and postoperative scores. In the literature to date, only one study with a prospective, controlled design has been identified in which self-esteem was measured at both timepoints.[72] In this study, it was found that women undergoing labiaplasty will experience improved self-esteem pertaining to genital appearance postoperatively, but there will be no change in one's general psychological well-being. Thus, we must consider study methodologies when interpreting positive results so as to not inflate the findings.

Although esthetic genital surgery may not necessarily improve overall psychological well-being, improvement in one's self-esteem as it pertains to appearance has the potential to improve one's sexual experience.[17] This finding has been supported in the esthetic surgery literature where women undergoing nongenital esthetic procedures, namely breast augmentation and body contouring, reported improvements in sexual satisfaction and an enhanced ability to achieve orgasm postoperatively.[73] Further, more than half of the women in this study testified to an enhancement of their partner's sex life on account of the powerful psychosexual effect of esthetic surgery on appearance-related self-esteem. These findings testify to inability to separate image and function.

Concerns and Recommendations

In the face of ongoing discrimination in the health care setting and public shame, patients with self-perceived anomalies will often turn to the mass media for information, which permits both a sense of community when desired and anonymity when needed. Unlike peer-reviewed journal articles, the media does not review the qualifications of the individuals claiming to be "experts," nor does it screen for legitimacy of disseminated information. In an evolving field with multiple specialties now offering esthetic genital surgery with little interdisciplinary communication, misinformation is highly prevalent and the general public's ability to recognize what is normal or critically evaluate the reliability of sources are matters for debate.[1,20,34,74,75]

There is a need for higher quality patient education, including images, videos, and clearer guidelines on content creation. A review of online advertisements for esthetic genital surgery found that the "before" images of female genitalia represented larger labia, albeit within a normal range, and were correlated with "ugliness," "odor," and "irritation." In contrast, the "after" images generally showed a "homogenized vulval appearance" without protrusion of the labia minora.[76] As we strive to foster and improve body image as plastic surgeons, it is imperative that we amplify body positivity and promote realistic, non-idealized images without pejorative references.

Studies suggest patient education regarding diversity of female genital appearance can improve female genital self-image.[77] In addition, we recommend characterizing preoperative and postoperative symptoms using a validated tool, such as the Female Sexual Function Index to assess sexual function, the Genital Appearance Satisfaction scale to evaluate genital self-image, and the Cosmetic Procedures Screening for Labiaplasty to distinguish between patients with and without BDD.[25,78] Postoperative scores should be determined not earlier than 6 months postoperatively to avoid the effect that cognitive dissonance may have on patient-reported outcomes.[79]

The media provides an opportunity to reach most, if not all, women considering esthetic genital surgery. Through the media, plastic surgeons, given their training and expertise, are in a unique position to educate not only their patients about the expectations and safety of esthetic genital surgery but also the public at large.

DISCUSSION
Controversies

Paradoxically, there is a social conscience to oppose esthetic genital surgery, yet accept other cosmetic procedures, such as augmentation mammoplasty.[20] Even within the realm of esthetic genital appearance, a discrepancy exists between surgical and nonsurgical treatment modalities, such that the public tends to support nonsurgical practices that involve waxing and "vajacials," yet dismiss surgical revision despite the same overarching goal.

Adding further controversy, in 2007, the American College of Obstetricians and Gynecologists released a comment in which they referred to esthetic genital procedures as being "untenable," as they pose substantial risk without medical benefit.[80] These opinions were restated in 2020, albeit with softer language, emphasizing that there is limited data on the risks and benefits of esthetic genital procedures.[81]

Future Directions

Within reason, a plastic surgeon's scope of practice is at the whim of what society wants. Historically, all patients with congenital adrenal hyperplasia underwent some form of feminizing genitoplasty in the newborn period.[82] More recently, however, families and providers are starting to delay reconstructive surgery until the patient can participate in the discussion of their own care.[83] Although increasing patient autonomy is noble and important, it must be taken with caution in vulnerable populations.

In the realm of esthetic genital surgery, there has been a rising subset of adolescent patients seeking modification, and we expect this number to continue to increase. According to the American Society for Aesthetic Plastic Surgery, there were 469 patients aged 18 years and younger who underwent labiaplasty in 2017, representing a 196% increase from 2014.[84] Although traditionally you do not perform a rhinoplasty until puberty is complete due to the potential growth of the facial skeleton, asymmetric development of the external genitalia may occur and continue throughout adolescence until the vagina finalizes its form.[8] A particular concern of working with adolescents is that they may not fully understand the risks, benefits, and long-term implications.

There has also been a rise in gender nonconforming patients seeking modification. Akin to adolescent women desiring labiaplasty, every intervention has potential ramifications down the road, and at this point, it is unclear to what end are genital esthetics. Nonetheless, plastic surgeons are and will continue to adapt to needs and issues as they arise. Being at the forefront of change is never easy, although it is necessary and worthwhile should these novel techniques improve the lives and well-being of our patients.

CLINICS CARE POINTS

- Genital self-image is the perception of one's own genital appearance and is influenced by the media, social and cultural expectations, and childbearing.

- Esthetic genital surgery is associated with high patient satisfaction and seems to have a positive effect on self-esteem as it pertains to one's genital appearance (not necessarily one's general psychological well-being). However, most of the studies fail to use a validated, quantitative methodology to assess outcomes.

- Three validated tools to characterize a patient's genital self-image exist. It is recommended that validated tools be used preoperatively on all patients considering esthetic genital surgery and no earlier than 6 months postoperatively.

DISCLOSURE

The authors have no commercial or financial conflicts of interest to disclose.

REFERENCES

1. Dogan O, Yassa M. Major motivators and sociodemographic features of women undergoing labiaplasty. Aesthet Surg J 2019;39(12):NP517–27.
2. Sorice SC, Li AY, Canales FL, et al. Why women request labiaplasty. Plast Reconstr Surg 2017; 139(4):856–63.
3. Veale D, Eshkevari E, Ellison N, et al. Psychological characteristics and motivation of women seeking labiaplasty. Psychol Med 2014;44(3):555–66.
4. Sharp G, Tiggemann M, Mattiske J. Factors that influence the decision to undergo labiaplasty: media, relationships, and psychological well-being. Aesthet Surg J 2016;36(4):469–78.
5. Crouch NS, Deans R, Michala L, et al. Clinical characteristics of well women seeking labial reduction surgery: a prospective study. BJOG 2011;118(12): 1507–10.
6. Goodman MP, Placik OJ, Benson RH, et al. A large multicenter outcome study of female genital plastic surgery. J Sex Med 2010;7(4 Pt 1):1565–77.
7. Zwier S. What motivates her": motivations for considering labial reduction surgery as recounted on women's online communities and surgeons' websites. Sex Med 2014;2(1):16–23.

8. Sharp G, Mattiske J, Vale KI. Motivations, expectations, and experiences of labiaplasty: a qualitative study. Aesthet Surg J 2016;36(8):920–8.
9. Phillips KA. The presentation of body dysmorphic disorder in medical settings. Prim Psychiatry 2006; 13(7):51–9.
10. Faravelli C, Salvatori S, Galassi F, et al. Epidemiology of somatoform disorders: a community survey in Florence. Soc Psychiatry Psychiatr Epidemiol 1997;32(1):24–9.
11. Castle DJ, Phillips KA, Dufresne RG. Body dysmorphic disorder and cosmetic dermatology: more than skin deep. J Cosmet Dermatol 2004;3(2): 99–103.
12. Castle DJ, Honigman RJ, Phillips KA. Does cosmetic surgery improve psychosocial wellbeing? Med J Aust 2002;176(12):601–4.
13. Turini T, Weck Roxo AC, Serra-Guimarães F, et al. The impact of labiaplasty on sexuality. Plast Reconstr Surg 2018;141(1):87–92.
14. Al-Jumah MM, Al-Wailiy SK, Al-Badr A. Satisfaction survey of women after cosmetic genital procedures: a cross-sectional study from Saudi Arabia. Aesthet Surg J Open Forum 2021;3(1):ojaa048.
15. Goodman MP. Female genital cosmetic and plastic surgery: a review. J Sex Med 2011;8(6):1813–25.
16. Lembo F, Cecchino LR, Parisi D, et al. What the women want". an overview on labiaplasty: function and beauty researched with an aesthetic gynecological procedure. RMGO 2020;5(4):1–6.
17. Goodman MP, Placik OJ, Matlock DL, et al. Evaluation of body image and sexual satisfaction in women undergoing female genital plastic/cosmetic surgery. Aesthet Surg J 2016;36(9):1048–57.
18. Phillips KA, Hollander E, Rasmussen SA, et al. A severity rating scale for body dysmorphic disorder: development, reliability, and validity of a modified version of the Yale-Brown Obsessive Compulsive Scale. Psychopharmacol Bull 1997; 33(1):17–22.
19. Honoré LH, O'Hara KE. Benign enlargement of the labia minora: report of two cases. Eur J Obstet Gynecol Reprod Biol 1978;8(2):61–4.
20. Sasson DC, Hamori CA, Placik OJ. Labiaplasty: the stigma persists. Aesthet Surg J 2022;42(6):638–43.
21. Runacres SA, Wood PL. Cosmetic labiaplasty in an adolescent population. J Pediatr Adolesc Gynecol 2016;29(3):218–22.
22. Widschwendter A, Riedl D, Freidhager K, et al. Perception of labial size and objective measurements-is there a correlation? A cross-sectional study in a cohort not seeking labiaplasty. J Sex Med 2020;17(3):461–9. https://doi.org/10.1016/j.jsxm.2019.11.272.
23. Herbenick D, Reece M. Development and validation of the female genital self-image scale. J Sex Med 2010;7(5):1822–30.

24. Veale D, Eshkevari E, Ellison N, et al. A comparison of risk factors for women seeking labiaplasty compared to those not seeking labiaplasty. Body Image 2014;11(1):57–62.

25. Veale D, Eshkevari E, Ellison N, et al. Validation of genital appearance satisfaction scale and the cosmetic procedure screening scale for women seeking labiaplasty. J Psychosom Obstet Gynaecol 2013;34(1):46–52.

26. Austin RE, Lista F, Vastis P-G, et al. Posterior vaginoplasty with perineoplasty: a canadian experience with vaginal tightening surgery. Aesthet Surg J Open Forum 2019;1(4):ojz030.

27. Janssen DF. First stirrings: cultural notes on orgasm, ejaculation, and wet dreams. J Sex Res 2007;44(2):122–34.

28. How many people use social media in 2021? (65+ statistics). Available at: https://backlinko.com/social-media-users. Accessed December 10, 2021.

29. Usage of social media as a news source worldwide 2021 | Statista. Available at: https://www.statista.com/statistics/718019/social-media-news-source/. Accessed December 10, 2021.

30. Millennials news consumption sources in the U.S. 2021 | Statista. Available at: https://www.statista.com/statistics/1010456/united-states-millennials-news-consumption/. Accessed December 10, 2021.

31. Schick VR, Rima BN, Calabrese SK. Evulvalution: the portrayal of women's external genitalia and physique across time and the current barbie doll ideals. J Sex Res 2011;48(1):74–81.

32. Sharp G, Tiggemann M, Mattiske J. Predictors of consideration of labiaplasty: an extension of the tripartite influence model of beauty ideals. Psychol Women Q 2015;39(2):182–93.

33. Hamilton EA, Mintz L, Kashubeck-West S. Predictors of media effects on body dissatisfaction in european american women. Sex Roles 2007;56(5–6):397–402.

34. Moran C, Lee C. What's normal? Influencing women's perceptions of normal genitalia: an experiment involving exposure to modified and nonmodified images. BJOG 2014;121(6):761–6.

35. Michala L. The adolescent and genital dissatisfaction. Clin Obstet Gynecol 2020;63(3):528–35. https://doi.org/10.1097/GRF.0000000000000522.

36. Müllerová J, Weiss P. Plastic surgery in gynaecology: factors affecting women's decision to undergo labiaplasty. Mind the risk of body dysmorphic disorder: a review. J Women Aging 2020;32(3):241–58.

37. Glazener CM. Sexual function after childbirth: women's experiences, persistent morbidity and lack of professional recognition. Br J Obstet Gynaecol 1997;104(3):330–5.

38. Barrett G, Pendry E, Peacock J, et al. Women's sexual health after childbirth. BJOG 2000;107(2):186–95.

39. Chang S-R, Chen K-H, Ho H-N, et al. Depressive symptoms, pain, and sexual dysfunction over the first year following vaginal or cesarean delivery: a prospective longitudinal study. Int J Nurs Stud 2015;52(9):1433–44.

40. Jawed-Wessel S, Herbenick D, Schick V. The relationship between body image, female genital self-image, and sexual function among first-time mothers. J Sex Marital Ther 2017;43(7):618–32.

41. Mullinax M, Herbenick D, Schick V, et al. In their own words: a qualitative content analysis of women's and men's preferences for women's genitals. Sex Educ 2015;15(4):421–36.

42. ClinicalKey. Available at: https://www.clinicalkey.com/nursing/#!/content/playContent/1-s2.0-S1751485117301587?returnurl=https%3A%2F%2Flinkinghub.elsevier.com%2Fretrieve%2Fpii%2FS1751485117301587%3Fshowall%3Dtrue&referrer=https%3A%2F%2Fpubmed.ncbi.nlm.nih.gov%2F. Accessed December 14, 2021.

43. Herbenick D, Schick V, Reece M, et al. Pubic hair removal among women in the United States: prevalence, methods, and characteristics. J Sex Med 2010;7(10):3322–30. https://doi.org/10.1111/j.1743-6109.2010.01935.x.

44. Female genital mutilation (FGM) statistics - UNICEF data. Available at: https://data.unicef.org/topic/child-protection/female-genital-mutilation/. Accessed June 14, 2021.

45. Sharif Mohamed F, Wild V, Earp BD, et al. Clitoral reconstruction after female genital mutilation/cutting: a review of surgical techniques and ethical debate. J Sex Med 2020;17(3):531–42.

46. Berg RC, Taraldsen S, Said MA, et al. Reasons for and experiences with surgical interventions for female genital mutilation/cutting (FGM/C): a systematic review. J Sex Med 2017;14(8):977–90.

47. Foldès P, Cuzin B, Andro A. Reconstructive surgery after female genital mutilation: a prospective cohort study. Lancet 2012;380(9837):134–41.

48. Merckelbagh HM, Nicolas MN, Piketty MP, et al. [Assessment of a multidisciplinary care for 169 excised women with an initial reconstructive surgery project]. Gynecol Obstet Fertil 2015;43(10):633–9.

49. Abramowicz S, Oden S, Dietrich G, et al. [Anatomic, functional and identity results after clitoris transposition]. J Gynecol Obstet Biol Reprod (Paris) 2016;45(8):963–71.

50. Ouédraogo CMR, Madzou S, Touré B, et al. [Practice of reconstructive plastic surgery of the clitoris after genital mutilation in Burkina Faso. Report of 94 cases]. Ann Chir Plast Esthet 2013;58(3):208–15.

51. Safari F. A qualitative study of women's lived experience after deinfibulation in the UK. Midwifery 2013;29(2):154–8.

52. Byrd-Bredbenner C, Murray J, Schlussel YR. Temporal changes in anthropometric measurements of idealized females and young women in general. Women Health 2005;41(2):13–30.

53. Plastic surgery statistics | american society of plastic surgeons. Available at: https://www.plasticsurgery.org/news/plastic-surgery-statistics. Accessed November 30, 2021.

54. Statistics. Available at: https://www.surgery.org/media/statistics. Accessed December 12, 2021.

55. Placik OJ, Arkins JP. Plastic surgery trends parallel Playboy magazine: the pudenda preoccupation. Aesthet Surg J 2014;34(7):1083–90.

56. Hersant B, Meningaud J-P. Commentary on: labiaplasty: the stigma persists. Aesthet Surg J 2022; 42(6):647–8. https://doi.org/10.1093/asj/sjab372.

57. Rouzier R, Louis-Sylvestre C, Paniel BJ, et al. Hypertrophy of labia minora: experience with 163 reductions. Am J Obstet Gynecol 2000;182(1 Pt 1):35–40.

58. Alter GJ. Aesthetic labia minora and clitoral hood reduction using extended central wedge resection. Plast Reconstr Surg 2008;122(6):1780–9.

59. Gress S. Composite reduction labiaplasty. Aesthet Plast Surg 2013;37(4):674–83.

60. Veale D, Naismith I, Eshkevari E, et al. Psychosexual outcome after labiaplasty: a prospective case-comparison study. Int Urogynecol J 2014;25(6): 831–9.

61. Sharp G, Maynard P, Hudaib A-R, et al. Do genital cosmetic procedures improve women's self-esteem? A systematic review and meta-analysis. Aesthet Surg J 2020;40(10):1143–51.

62. Sorice-Virk S, Li AY, Canales FL, et al. Comparison of patient symptomatology before and after labiaplasty. Plast Reconstr Surg 2020;146(3):526–36.

63. Kelishadi SS, Omar R, Herring N, et al. The safe labiaplasty: a study of nerve density in labia minora and its implications. Aesthet Surg J 2016;36(6): 705–9.

64. Hunter JG. Labia minora, labia majora, and clitoral hood alteration: experience-based recommendations. Aesthet Surg J 2016;36(1):71–9.

65. Bucknor A, Chen AD, Egeler S, et al. Labiaplasty: indications and predictors of postoperative sequelae in 451 consecutive cases. Aesthet Surg J 2018; 38(6):644–53.

66. Shahghaibi S, Faizi S, Gharibi F. Effect of colporrhaphy on the Sexual Dysfunction of women with pelvic organ prolapsed. Pak J Med Sci Q 2013;29(1): 157–60.

67. Ulubay M, Keskin U, Fidan U, et al. Safety, efficiency, and outcomes of perineoplasty: treatment of the sensation of a wide vagina. Biomed Res Int 2016; 2016:2495105.

68. Dobbeleir JMLCL, Landuyt KV, Monstrey SJ. Aesthetic surgery of the female genitalia. Semin Plast Surg 2011;25(2):130–41.

69. Gonzalez F, Dass D, Almeida B. Custom flask labiaplasty. Ann Plast Surg 2015;75(3):266–71.

70. Ouar N, Guillier D, Moris V, et al. [Postoperative complications of labia minora reduction. Comparative study between wedge and edge resection]. Ann Chir Plast Esthet 2017;62(3):219–23.

71. Lista F, Mistry BD, Singh Y, et al. The safety of aesthetic labiaplasty: a plastic surgery experience. Aesthet Surg J 2015;35(6):689–95.

72. Sharp G, Tiggemann M, Mattiske J. Psychological outcomes of labiaplasty: a prospective study. Plast Reconstr Surg 2016;138(6):1202–9.

73. Stofman GM, Neavin TS, Ramineni PM, et al. Better sex from the knife? An intimate look at the effects of cosmetic surgery on sexual practices. Aesthet Surg J 2006;26(1):12–7.

74. Braun V. Female genital cosmetic surgery: a critical review of current knowledge and contemporary debates. J Womens Health (Larchmt) 2010;19(7):1393–407.

75. Cosmetic gynecology and the elusive quest for the "perfect" vagina. Obstet Gynecol 2012;119(6): 1083–4.

76. Liao L-M, Taghinejadi N, Creighton SM. An analysis of the content and clinical implications of online advertisements for female genital cosmetic surgery. BMJ Open 2012;2(6). https://doi.org/10.1136/bmjopen-2012-001908.

77. Fernando AN, Sharp G. Genital self-image in adolescent girls: the effectiveness of a brief educational video. Body Image 2020;35:75–83.

78. Isidori AM, Pozza C, Esposito K, et al. Development and validation of a 6-item version of the female sexual function index (FSFI) as a diagnostic tool for female sexual dysfunction. J Sex Med 2010;7(3): 1139–46.

79. Sharp G, Maynard P, Hamori CA, et al. Measuring quality of life in female genital cosmetic procedure patients: a systematic review of patient-reported outcome measures. Aesthet Surg J 2020;40(3): 311–8.

80. Committee on Gynecologic Practice, American College of Obstetricians and Gynecologists. ACOG Committee Opinion No, 378. Vaginal "rejuvenation" and cosmetic vaginal procedures. Obstet Gynecol 2007;110(3):737–8.

81. Elective female genital cosmetic surgery: ACOG committee opinion summary, number 795. Obstet Gynecol 2020;135(1):249–50.

82. Dwiggins M, Brookner B, Fowler K, et al. Multidimensional aspects of female sexual function in congenital adrenal hyperplasia: a case-control study. J Endocr Soc 2020;4(11):bvaa131.

83. Chawla R, Rutter M, Green J, et al. Care of the adolescent patient with congenital adrenal hyperplasia: special considerations, shared decision making, and transition. Semin Pediatr Surg 2019; 28(5):150845.

84. Cosmetic surgery national data bank statistics. Aesthet Surg J 2018;38(suppl_3):1–24.

UNITED STATES POSTAL SERVICE ®

Statement of Ownership, Management, and Circulation (All Periodicals Publications Except Requester Publications)

1. Publication Title	2. Publication Number	3. Filing Date
CLINICS IN PLASTIC SURGERY	006 – 530	9/18/2022

4. Issue Frequency	5. Number of Issues Published Annually	6. Annual Subscription Price
JAN, APR, JUL, OCT	4	$548.00

7. Complete Mailing Address of Known Office of Publication (Not printer) (Street, city, county, state, and ZIP+4®)

ELSEVIER INC.
230 Park Avenue, Suite 800
New York, NY 10169

Contact Person
Malathi Samayan

Telephone (Include area code)
91-44-4299-4507

8. Complete Mailing Address of Headquarters or General Business Office of Publisher (Not printer)

ELSEVIER INC.
230 Park Avenue, Suite 800
New York, NY 10169

9. Full Names and Complete Mailing Addresses of Publisher, Editor, and Managing Editor (Do not leave blank)

Publisher (Name and complete mailing address)

DOLORES MELONI, ELSEVIER INC.
1600 JOHN F KENNEDY BLVD. SUITE 1800
PHILADELPHIA, PA 19103-2899

Editor (Name and complete mailing address)

STACY EASTMAN, ELSEVIER INC.
1600 JOHN F KENNEDY BLVD. SUITE 1800
PHILADELPHIA, PA 19103-2899

Managing Editor (Name and complete mailing address)

PATRICK MANLEY, ELSEVIER INC.
1600 JOHN F KENNEDY BLVD. SUITE 1800
PHILADELPHIA, PA 19103-2899

10. Owner (Do not leave blank. If the publication is owned by a corporation, give the name and address of the corporation immediately followed by the names and addresses of all stockholders owning or holding 1 percent or more of the total amount of stock. If not owned by a corporation, give the names and addresses of the individual owners. If owned by a partnership or other unincorporated firm, give its name and address as well as those of each individual owner. If the publication is published by a nonprofit organization, give its name and address.)

Full Name	Complete Mailing Address
WHOLLY OWNED SUBSIDIARY OF REED/ELSEVIER, US HOLDINGS	1600 JOHN F KENNEDY BLVD. SUITE 1800 PHILADELPHIA, PA 19103-2899

11. Known Bondholders, Mortgagees, and Other Security Holders Owning or Holding 1 Percent or More of Total Amount of Bonds, Mortgages, or Other Securities. If none, check box ► ☐ None

Full Name	Complete Mailing Address
N/A	

12. Tax Status (For completion by nonprofit organizations authorized to mail at nonprofit rates) (Check one)
The purpose, function, and nonprofit status of this organization and the exempt status for federal income tax purposes:
☒ Has Not Changed During Preceding 12 Months
☐ Has Changed During Preceding 12 Months (Publisher must submit explanation of change with this statement)

PS Form 3526, July 2014 [Page 1 of 4 (see instructions page 4)] PSN: 7530-01-000-9931 PRIVACY NOTICE: See our privacy policy on www.usps.com.

---

13. Publication Title	14. Issue Date for Circulation Data Below
CLINICS IN PLASTIC SURGERY	JULY 2022

15. Extent and Nature of Circulation			Average No. Copies Each Issue During Preceding 12 Months	No. Copies of Single Issue Published Nearest to Filing Date
a. Total Number of Copies (Net press run)			268	235
b. Paid Circulation (By Mail and Outside the Mail)	(1)	Mailed Outside-County Paid Subscriptions Stated on PS Form 3541 (Include paid distribution above nominal rate, advertiser's proof copies, and exchange copies)	131	116
	(2)	Mailed In-County Paid Subscriptions Stated on PS Form 3541 (Include paid distribution above nominal rate, advertiser's proof copies, and exchange copies)	0	0
	(3)	Paid Distribution Outside the Mails Including Sales Through Dealers and Carriers, Street Vendors, Counter Sales, and Other Paid Distribution Outside USPS®	83	73
	(4)	Paid Distribution by Other Classes of Mail Through the USPS (e.g., First-Class Mail®)	0	0
c. Total Paid Distribution (Sum of 15b (1), (2), (3), and (4))		►	214	189
d. Free or Nominal Rate Distribution (By Mail and Outside the Mail)	(1)	Free or Nominal Rate Outside-County Copies included on PS Form 3541	33	25
	(2)	Free or Nominal Rate In-County Copies Included on PS Form 3541	0	0
	(3)	Free or Nominal Rate Copies Mailed at Other Classes Through the USPS (e.g., First-Class Mail)	0	0
	(4)	Free or Nominal Rate Distribution Outside the Mail (Carriers or other means)	0	0
e. Total Free or Nominal Rate Distribution (Sum of 15d (1), (2), (3) and (4))		►	33	25
f. Total Distribution (Sum of 15c and 15e)		►	247	214
g. Copies not Distributed (See Instructions to Publishers #4 (page #3))		►	21	21
h. Total (Sum of 15f and g)		►	268	235
i. Percent Paid (15c divided by 15f times 100)		►	86.63%	88.31%

* If you are claiming electronic copies, go to line 16 on page 3. If you are not claiming electronic copies, skip to line 17 on page 3.

PS Form 3526, July 2014 (Page 2 of 4)

16. Electronic Copy Circulation	Average No. Copies Each Issue During Preceding 12 Months	No. Copies of Single Issue Published Nearest to Filing Date
a. Paid Electronic Copies ►		
b. Total Paid Print Copies (Line 15c) + Paid Electronic Copies (Line 16a) ►		
c. Total Print Distribution (Line 15f) + Paid Electronic Copies (Line 16a) ►		
d. Percent Paid (Both Print & Electronic Copies) (16b divided by 16c × 100) ►		

☒ I certify that 50% of all my distributed copies (electronic and print) are paid above a nominal price.

17. Publication of Statement of Ownership

☒ If the publication is a general publication, publication of this statement is required. Will be printed in the OCTOBER 2022 issue of this publication. ☐ Publication not required.

18. Signature and Title of Editor, Publisher, Business Manager, or Owner

Malathi Samayan Date 9/18/2022

Malathi Samayan - Distribution Controller

I certify that all information furnished on this form is true and complete. I understand that anyone who furnishes false or misleading information on this form or who omits material or information requested on the form may be subject to criminal sanctions (including fines and imprisonment) and/or civil sanctions (including civil penalties).

PS Form 3526, July 2014 (Page 3 of 4) PRIVACY NOTICE: See our privacy policy on www.usps.com.

Moving?

Make sure your subscription moves with you!

To notify us of your new address, find your **Clinics Account Number** (located on your mailing label above your name), and contact customer service at:

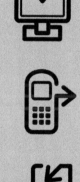

Email: journalscustomerservice-usa@elsevier.com

800-654-2452 (subscribers in the U.S. & Canada)
314-447-8871 (subscribers outside of the U.S. & Canada)

Fax number: 314-447-8029

Elsevier Health Sciences Division
Subscription Customer Service
3251 Riverport Lane
Maryland Heights, MO 63043

Printed and bound by CPI Group (UK) Ltd, Croydon, CR0 4YY

11/05/2025

01866593-0001